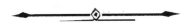

ISBN 978-0-331-10066-2
PIBN 11014157

This book is a reproduction of an important historical work. Forgotten Books uses state-of-the-art technology to digitally reconstruct the work, preserving the original format whilst repairing imperfections present in the aged copy. In rare cases, an imperfection in the original, such as a blemish or missing page, may be replicated in our edition. We do, however, repair the vast majority of imperfections successfully; any imperfections that remain are intentionally left to preserve the state of such historical works.

THE

NATURE, CAUSES, SYMPTOMS AND CURE

OF DISEASES OF THE

THROAT AND LUNGS.

THE DIFFERENCE BETWEEN

RON̲ ̲ITIS, CLERGYMAN'S SORE THROAT,

AND

CONSUMPTION;

TH A NEW AND CERTAIN METHOD OF ASCERTAINING THE EXISTENCE OF THIS LAST NAMED DISEASE, IN ITS EARLIEST STAGES, WITH NUMEROUS ILLUSTRATIONS BY FACTS AND CASES.

By W. W. Hall, A. M., M. D.

'ARTICULAR NOTICE.—Hereafter, my Office will be open from May 20th to November ., at the Corner of Fourth and Vine streets, CINCINNATI; and from November 1st, to May th, of each year, at 127 Canal Street, Corner of Baronne Street, NEW ORLEANS.
Strangers may save themselves much time and trouble and disappointment, by attend- ; to this precaution, as there are several practitioners of a similar name, or near the ne locality, in both cities.
The full bound edition of this publication, (220 pages, bound in cloth, fifth edition, th engravings,) is sold by J. B. STEELE, 14 Camp Street NEW ORLEANS, and J. D. IORPE, Bookseller, 12, Fourth Street, CINCINNATI, where directions us to the ality of my Office, will be courteously given.

PRICE, TWENTY-FIVE CENTS.

SOLD BY:—J. B. STEELE, 14, *Camp street, New Orleans,*
J. D. THORPE, 12, *West Fourth street, Cincinnati,*
BURGESS & STRINGER, 222, *Broadway New York,*.
MOORE & Co., 193, *Chesnut street, Philadelphia,*
WATERS, 244, *Market street, Baltimore,*
JAS. FRENCH, 78, *Washington street, Boston,*
A. HEAD, *Charleston,*
FRANK TAYLOR, *Washington,*
C. C. CLEAVES, *Memphis,*
BOULLEMET, *Mobile,*
SKILLMAN, *Opposite Planters' House, St. Louis,*
NOBLE, 66, *Fourth street, Louisville,*
M. P. MORSE, *Pittsburgh.*

CINCINNATI:

PRINTED BY JOHN D. THORPE, 12, WEST FOURTH STREET.
1850.

CLERGYMAN'S SORE THROAT.

D_R. HALL's LETTER TO REV. M. M. ———, OF OHIO.

CINCINNATI. October 15th, 1847.

Reverend and Dear Sir :—As you are now engaged in preaching every day, although the affection of your throat and breast had compelled you for some time to abandon public speaking, I yield to the inquiries made in your letter.

What is commonly called Bronchitis, (pronounced *Bron-kee-tis*,) Clergyman's Sore Throat, Throat Consumption. &c., is *Chronic Laryngitis*—that is inflammation, and finally, ulceration of the voice-making organs, which are situated in the region of Adam's apple : it is brought on by over-exertion of the voice ; by sudden changes from hot to cold air, or the reverse ; by the application of cold, or dampness to any part of the body. It comes on by a pricking sensation in swallowing, or in suddenly turning the head ; sometimes a heavy, dull aching feeling is experienced about the sides of Adam's apple, or pain is felt on slight pressure at those points, or in front. In other cases, there is no feeling of pain or soreness, but a constant disposition to hawk or swallow—an instinctive effort to clear the throat before speaking to a person. There is often no cough at all ; but in clearing the throat, a pearly, tough, ropy, sticky substance is brought away, with more or less difficulty. When a yellowish matter is brought up with a simple hem, an ulcer is present, and there is imminent danger of a total and irrecoverable loss of voice, and of life. But the most uniform symptom of the beginning of this hitherto fatal form of disease, is a greater or less degree of hoarseness, huskiness or other impairment of the voice, lasting for several weeks in succession.

When a person cannot swallow food or cold water without coughing, and sometimes driving it back through the nose, ulcers are already formed, or forming : this symptom appears in the latter stages of the disease.

The mode of cure is one of the most admirable discoveries of modern times, because

1. No internal medicine is necessary, if the general health be good.
2. The patient is not confined to the house for a single hour in the day.
3. The remedy is prompt, safe and sure.

Ordinarily, under proper treatment, ulcers begin to heal within thirty-six hours ; and unless the case be an aggravated one, the voice becomes clearer after three or four applications.

I knew a young lady from the South, aged nineteen, who had not spoken above a whisper for nine months ; after the third application, she rose from her chair, bathed in tears, expressing her gratitude and joy in a clear and natural tone.

A sugar planter came to my office, with a voice so deranged, that I could only hear by placing my cheek to his lips. He had applied to Professor ———, of the——Medical School in another State, who thought he could restore his voice in three days. The neck was extensively blistered, and twelve leeches were applied to the throat at one time. At the end of three weeks he was in every way weaker and worse. He came to me, and on the eighth day after, his voice was clear and strong ; and he left my office the happiest man I had seen for many months. No internal medicine was given in this case, except a common anodyne, to allay the nervous irritability of the system, and a tonic to restore the nervous power to the parts more immediately affected. The main treatment was by local applications, directly to the organs of voice.

The mode of cure is easily described—it is the daily application, without pain, of medicinal agents to the voice-making organs, and *below them*, when necessary, as far down the windpipe as the bottom of the neck.—When, by unwise delays, the ulceration has been allowed to extend itself below that point

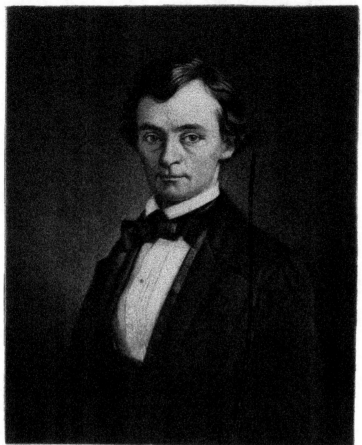

Engᵈ by W. Warner from a Daguerreotype by McClees & Germon.

W. W. Hall

Middleton Printer

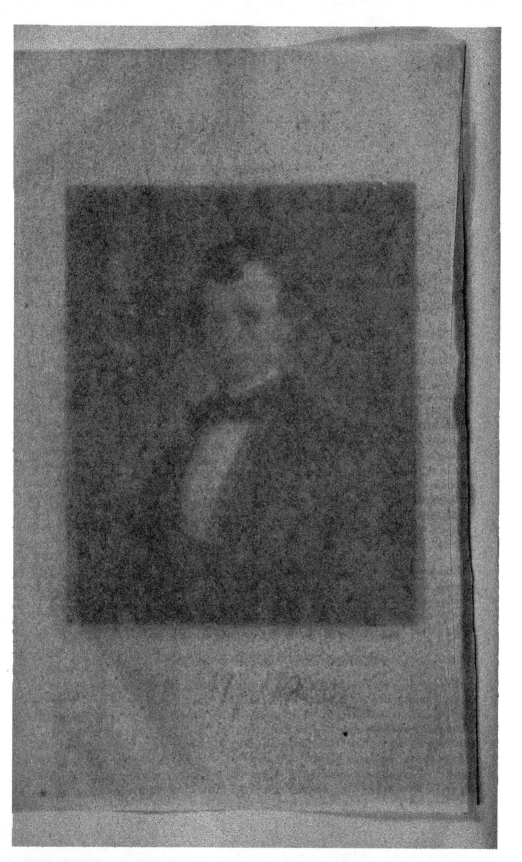

DR. HALL

ON DISEASES OF THE

THROAT AND LUNGS.

" It is adverse to the interests of humanity to consider any disease incurable."
SIR CHARLES SCUDAMORE.

" Consumption is clearly Scrofula, and admits of only one mode of cure."
JOHN HUNTER.

" I have no doubt but that there is a specific for Consumption." DR. STOKES.

" Its perfect cure is demonstrable." DR. CARSWELL.

FOR CONFIRMED CONSUMPTION I KNOW OF NO CURE. THE AUTHOR.

Before the lungs begin to decay, judicious treatment will generally restore to health with little or no internal medicine. I use no secret remedies nor patent contrivances for the alleviation of human suffering. THE AUTHOR.

No educated physician of respectability and eminence, in Europe or America, will perhaps deny, if he has had any considerable experience in the treatment of consumptive diseases, that when the lungs are in a state of decay, viz., when persons are in the latter stages of consumption the disease is sometimes permanently arrested, and the person dies years afterwards of a totally different malady. While this is certainly true, it is the author's opinion, that such a result in any given case is seldom to be hoped for, unless in an iron constitution, and ought never to be promised.

WHAT IS CONSUMPTION?

Consumption, commonly called a " Decline," and by physicians " Phthisis," is a gradual wasting away of the lungs, by which they become disorganized or rotten, and are spit out of the mouth in the shape of yellow matter, which, as the disease advances, usually sinks in water, and in three cases out of four, is, or has been. more or less tinged with blood at various intervals.

GENERAL SYMPTOMS OF CONSUMPTION.

It is not as extensively known as it ought to be, that, in the large majority of cases, Consumption begins with *a slight cough in the morning on getting up.* After a while it is perceived at night on going to bed; next, there is an occasional " coughing spell " sometime during the night; by this time there is a difficulty of breathing on any slightly unusual exercise, or in going up stairs, or ascending a hill; and the patient expresses himself, with some surprise, " Why, it never used to tire me so !" Next, there is occasional coughing after a full meal, and sometimes " casting up." Even before this, persons begin to feel weak, while there is an almost im.

A

perceptible thinning in flesh, and a gradual diminution in weight—harrassing cough, loose bowels, difficult breathing, swollen extremities, daily fever, and a miserable death! Miserable, because it is tedious, painful, and inevitable. How much I wish that the symptoms of this hateful disease were more generally studied and understood by my fellow-countrymen and country-women, that they might detect it, in its first insidious approaches, and be induced to apply at once for their arrest and their total eradication; for certain I am that, in very many instances, it could be accomplished.

SPECIAL SYMPTOMS OF CONSUMPTION.

Quick pulse, hacking cough, general weakness, restless sleep, variable appetite, irregular bowels, pains between the shoulder-blades behind.

INFALLIBLE SYMPTOMS OF CONSUMPTION.

Coughing night and day, flabby muscles, general debility, great shortness of breath on going up stairs, ascending a hill, or walking but a little fast, pulse always above one hundred for weeks together; drenching cold sweats towards morning; copious expectoration of yellow matter, sometimes bloody, or rusty colored.

FATAL SYMPTOMS OF CONSUMPTION.

I have never known a man get well of Consumption who had all the following symptoms: A weak, thready pulse, constantly over one hundred in a minute; breathes habitually, even when quiet, more than thirty times in a minute; habitual coughing, and casting up after meals; spitting up, during the day and night, masses of a thick yellowish stuff, no saliva with it, and which falls on the floor with distinct edges, not ragged edges, or if in water, sinks in half a minute; drenching night sweats; several passages from the bowels every day, very much like rice water, with painful griping; a dull, heavy, or crampy pain in some of the muscles of the arms or legs; swollen ankles; cannot swallow easily, especially liquids, which sometimes come back through the nose; partial loss of the use of the legs. Such a man must die of the Consumption within a month. It is impossible for it to be any thing else but Consumption.

HISTORY OF A CASE OF CONSUMPTION.

No two cases of this disease are precisely alike in every particular: yet, in general, the feelings and symptoms in its beginning, progress, and end, are as follows:

In nearly every case, Consumption begins with a slight, short, tickling cough in the morning; but as it occurs only now and then, and is so very slight that only one or two efforts at coughing are made on getting up, it is not noticed at this stage. after a while, this cough occurs occasionally during the day; it may be next observed on lying down at night, or some minutes after being in bed; a single cough or two; coming on quite suddenly, as if produced by a particle of dust in the throat, from the pillow or bedding. Soon the morning cough increases, and the night cough comes on regularly; damp weather, or a sudden spell of cold weather, increases it, and the person says he has "caught a cold, somehow or other;" but it does not go off of itself, like a cold used to do; it "hangs on," and is increased by every slight change in the moisture or temperature of the atmosphere. The patient now begins to think he had " better take something " for his cold. He might discover, however, by this time, that it does not affect him as a cold used to do ; for several years ago, when he took a cold, he remembered that it made him "feel bad all over ;" his appetite decreased ; his nose would run almost constantly ; occasioning a snuffling every few minutes, with a stopping up in the head ; and he would cough, and cough hard, any time during the day, spitting up more or less of heavy yellow matter ; and he describes himself as being " out of sorts ;" but the cold he now has is quite a different thing ; his head is not stopped up ; his nose does not run ; his appetite is quite good ; he does not feel bad at all ; he spits up no yellow matter during the day or night either ; but he has simply a dry, short, tickling cough, which keeps him from going to sleep when he first gets into bed at night ; and which comes on in the morning as soon as he gets up and begins to stir about ; and with the exception of this, when he goes to bed, and when he gets up, he says he " feels well enough," having no headache, no fever, no burning feeling about the nostrils, and repeats for the hundredth time, " if I could only get rid of this cough, I would be as well as I ever was in my life." He then determines to " take something." Every body has a prescription that cured such and such an one, who "had just such a cough, only worse and of longer duration, and it is so simple that it could not possibly hurt any one." Some of these do no good whatever ; others give relief, but soon appear not to have the desired effect, and something else is resorted to, with similar results. But long before this time, a practised observer will have noticed that other changes have been taking place ; because, every hour, the disease has been digging its way deep down into the vitals. The pulse is more rapid than natural, has more of a quick, threadlike, spiteful beat ; and too weak, besides ; the patient is more easily tired than formerly, especially in going up stairs, or walking up a hill or gentle ascent ; when he attempts to do any thing, he " gives out" sooner than he used to, causing him to have an occasional shortness of breath ; about this time, he finds occasionally that he cannot take a full long breath as formerly ; something seems to cut it short, leaving an unsatisfied feeling ; his friends observe that he is as lively as usual. and indeed more so ; he feels, and appears cheerful ; and is quick in his movements ; but before he does much, or walks far, he becomes very weak about the legs and knees ; and there is a great craving for a place to sit down upon, and rest awhile ; and if a sofa or bed is near, it feels at first so comfortable that he is inclined to stay there ; now and then, there is a feeling of weight in the breast, dull, heavy, or cold-like ; if he leans forward much, his breast gives way ; pains more or less transient, or permanent, are felt in some part of the chest ; often these are at the lower edge of the ribs ; there is now an occasional feverishness ; the bowels become costive and loose alternately ; sometimes the feet or hands, or both, burn very much ; at others, they are uncomfortably cold ; the patient begins to think that he is " falling off " some ; and turns to weighing himself with very unsatisfactory results ; he perceives that although his appetite is quite good, his food does not seem to do him as much good as formerly ; there is unusual thirstiness during some part of the day ; if the weather is but a little cool, he gets very chilly ; after awhile, chills frequently run all over the body, and along the spine, without any apparent cause ; an emotion of the mind, a drink of cold water, is sufficient to send a succession of chilly sensations all through the system ; while these symptoms are presenting themselves, the original cough, although sometimes better, has, in the main, become decidedly worse, and more annoying ; it comes on as soon as the patient goes to bed, and continues from ten or fifteen minutes to two hours, according to circumstances ; throwing the system into a nervous irritable condition ; effectually preventing sleep for half the night, perhaps, when he falls into a doze from mere exhaustion; and in the morning he wakes up, pale and wan and haggard, without seeming to have derived any benefit whatever from his repose; and weak and wretched as he feels, the morning cough now attacks him, hard and dry at first, but in a few minutes he is relieved, by bringing up more or less of yellow matter, mixed with something of a whitish, frothy, bubbly character; coughing comes on after meals, with heaving, and in some cases vomiting, although not specially-attended with sickness at the stomach. As the disease progresses, he emaciates more and more, the weakness of the lower limbs increases, the amount of yellow matter expectorated becomes greater from day to day, while the frothy substance is less; there is more or less of thirst or chilliness between breakfast and dinner, with decided fever in the afternoon, which subsides during the fore part of the night, and goes off towards morning with a copious, exhausting, and death-like sweat, carrying damps and chilliness to the very heart; these sweats are accompanied, or alternated, with frequent and thin, watery, light colored passages from the bowels, from two or three to a dozen or more in the twenty-four hours, attended sometimes with horrible griping pains in the bowels; at other times, there are dull pains in the muscles and bones of the limbs, occasionally almost insupportable; even yet the patient may keep about, and appear quite cheerful; but his steps are slow, measured, and careful; his body bent forward; his shoulders inclining upon the breast, and towards one another; if he sits down a moment or two, his legs are crossed, his arms laid across his thighs, pressing upon his breast by leaning forward, and thus throwing the whole strain and weight of the body upon it, hastening his death by imposing an unnatural and unnecessary weight on the struggling lungs, already enfeebled and wasted by disease; he begins now to feel best in bed, where he spends the greater portion of the twenty-four hours; his ankles swell, generally the left first, often extending to the feet and legs, sometimes painfully; he cannot walk with comfort; and soon his mother earth receives him to her bosom, where myriads of her weary children have gone, to be wasted with sickness no more!

WHAT ARE THE LUNGS?

They are to man what the "lights" are to animals; are made in the same way, and look like them, hanging on both sides of the breast, and reaching down as far as the sixth rib. They are divided into five bunches, called lobes, three of which are in the right and two in the left side. They may be compared to many thousands of small bladders, called air cells, united in one great neck, the windpipe. They have their root at the back-bone, between the shoulder blades, and from that they stick out forwards, not entirely unlike the extended wings of a bird. These little air cells have exceeding thin sides, and are of all sizes, from the twentieth down to the hundredth part of an inch in diameter. They are filled with air at every breath we draw in; and are comparatively emptied at every outbreathing. And this is their employment, unceasingly, from the first cry of infancy till the last effort of expiring nature. The foundation for consumption is not unfrequently laid by the sides of these air cells thickening and sticking, or even growing together, from the want of full breathing enough to keep them apart, or from high mucous excitement, from various causes.

WHAT CAUSES THE LUNGS TO CONSUME?

Tubercles form on, around, and among the air cells which constitute the lungs, ripen, rot, and eat them away.

WHAT ARE TUBERCLES?

They are small rounded masses, which, as they enlarge, often acquire the form of a tuberous root, such as the potatoe, garlic, tulip, &c., and hence called Tubercle. A single tubercle is a small, clear, shining, gray substance, dotted about among the lungs, usually roundish, but of all shapes; and in size from a pea down to invisibility. In the course of time it begins to ripen, by a little yellow spot appearing, usually in the centre, and gradually widens to the edges. The tubercle now softens, spreads, meets its neighbor tubercle half way; these join, and meet others which have joined, and all soften down into one yellow mass together; this is spit up by degrees, and the place it occupied is empty, and is called a cavity, excavation, not unlike that made by mice in cheese; small, if it holds a hazlenut, and very large when a goose-egg may lay in it. Tubercles ripen at different times, as apples on a tree; and this is the reason that consumptive persons have such frequent changes in their feelings, well to-day, or this week, and ill the next. In process of time, other excavations are made, and communicate with older ones; and in this way the lungs are burrowed out to a mere shell; the man speaks in a sepulchral, grave-like voice, which it makes one shudder to hear, and soon there are not lungs enough left to live upon, to keep him warm; and the fire of life goes out—forever.

WHAT CAUSES TUBERCLES?

Some persons are born with them. Weak, sickly persons, those who are dyspeptic, drunken, effeminate, *diseased*, who marry too young, almost always send tuberculous children into the world, and leave them the woful heritage of a constitution blasted at the root.

When persons are not born consumptive, they may become so in many ways; for whatever impairs the general health is capable of producing tubercles in a few weeks, by impoverishing the blood. Whatever can impoverish the blood can cause consumption; and whatever enriches the blood arrests and cures it.

The causes which more commonly operate in effecting this gradual and almost imperceptible undermining of the health, are insufficient or bad food; scanty clothing; living in cellars or other damp situations; injudicious use of calomel, quinine, or intoxicating drinks; protracted fever and ague; suppressions; profuse discharges, long continued grief, disappointments, worldly care; intense and extended mental effort; neglected colds and coughs; frequent resort to medicine for slight ailments; costiveness alone, or alternating with loose bowels; breathing impure air, or the heated atmosphere of factories, engine rooms, printing offices; frequent and sudden changes from heat to cold, or from a cold to a hot temperature, such as pilots, engineers, and clergymen are subject to; these, and many others, by gradually undermining the health, lay the foundation for that truly distressing disease.

HOW ARE TUBERCLES PRODUCED?

On the sides of the air cells already spoken of, many little blood vessels spread themselves about in every direction, as a vine spreads itself on the side of a wall; through these all the blood of the body passes many times a day, if there is nothing to hinder it in its progress, and choke them up. When that is the case, the extremely thin sides of these blood-bearing vessels may yield a little, but the clogging still going on, the thinnest part of the blood is pressed through its pores, or there is a vitiated secretion, which stands there, in the shape of a small, clear drop, with, possibly, the slightest tinge of red; this soon enlarges, hardens, and is a young tubercle, and this it is, which causes the dry, hacking cough in consumption, seeming to come on of itself, yet gives a timely and friendly warning, but gives it most frequently in vain. The mere existence of tubercles is not necessarily injurious; they are present in the lungs of thousands, of perhaps a majority of people to the close of life, without doing any appreciable injury. It may, in truth, be said, that all grown persons have tubercles to a greater or less extent; they are made fatal by bad colds, and weakening ailments; and these are occasioned by reckless exposure, and various kinds of intemperance, diet, drink, dress, indulgence of passions, &c.

WHAT DO TUBERCLES PRODUCE?

They give rise to various diseases, according to the part of the body in which they are located.

Tubercle in the Lungs is Consumption.
Tubercle in the Neck is King's Evil.
Tubercle in a Joint is White Swelling.
Tubercle in the Back-bone induces Spinal Disease.
Tubercle in the Loins is Lumbar Abscess.
Tubercle in the Hip is Hip Joint Disease.
Tubercle in the Nostrils of a horse is called Glanders.

Tubercle in the Abdomen is Nego Consumption, or Tabes Mesenterica, a general wasting away, without any special pain or other suffering; the patient eats and drinks as usual, but nothing that he eats seems to do him any good, gives him no strength; on the contrary, he gets weaker and weaker.

Children who have scabs and running sores about the nose ears, mouth, scalp, corners of the lips, &c., are Tuberculous.

Consumption, Scrofula, Struma, and Tubercles may be considered one and the same malady, modified by manifestation and locality.

WHAT IS BRONCHITIS?

If the reader remembers the symptoms of a common cold, and will imagine these symptoms to continue for weeks and months, then has he a correct idea of what Bronchitis really is.

Bronchitis is *Acute* when the symptoms of a common cold last for a few days; it is called *Chronic* when these symptoms are protracted through months; but common usage has abolished this scientific distinction, and applies the name of Bronchitis to the chronic form exclusively; while the acute form is universally designated as a " cold," or " bad cold." When, therefore, it is said that a man has Bronchitis, the chronic form is meant, Acute Bronchitis being expressed by the terms *Catarrh*, *Coryza, Common Cold*, all of which terms mean precisely the same thing, *common cold* being the English name, the others being of Greek origin.

At the bottom of the neck, in front, just at the top of the breast bone, there is a depression or hollow, and just below this the windpipe divides off into numerous branches, precisely like the trunk of a tree; these branches are called " Bronchi," a name given by the ancients, from the Greek word *Brecho*, which means to moisten, because they supposed that solids were introduced into the stomach by the gullet, but liquids by the branches of the windpipe; these branches are hollow, and are called Bronchial Tubes, whose insides have a very thin lining, over which innumerable blood vessels branch out, as a vine branches out on the side of a wall; when, by any means, these blood vessels have more blood in them than is natural, disease is constituted, and the name for such a state of things is *inflammation*, that is, *flamelike*, since wherever in the human body there is more blood than there ought to be, generally speaking, there is more redness and there is more heat, blood being warm and red as flames of fire are; but instead of using this long word *inflammation*, physicians adopt a shorter one of four letters, *itis*, and by attaching it to the name of any portion of the body it means inflammation of that portion of the body—that is, more blood in the small blood vessels of that part than there ought to be: hence, the word *itis* added to the name of the branches of the windpipe, makes the word Bronchitis, which, to express in full, we would have to say, " Too much blood in the small blood vessels which are spread over the lining of the inside of the branches of the windpipe." As many medical words end in *itis*, always pronounced as if written etis, the reader is requested to bear in mind that this expressive little word always means the same thing—that is, too much blood in the blood vessels of the part to which this word is attached; and if these parts were only designated by English names, common readers could have a clear understanding of all these forms of disease, without any difficulty. But, unfortunately, after all this trouble in endeavoring to tell the reader what Bronchitis is, in its true scientific meaning, I must say, that it has a very different signification in common conversation. Any cough, continuing for some time, is called Bronchitis, and that name is still applied, until the patient is dying, then it is called Consumption. If a man has a cough and gets well, he is said to have had *only Bronchitis*, but if he dies, it is written *"died of Consumption!"* I do not recollect, at this time, of ever having seen in an obituary notice, in a newspaper, the words, " died of Bronchitis." It is plain, then, that either the word is improperly used, or that Bronchitis never kills. The true state of the case is simply this: Bronchitis is a less terrifying name for Consumption, adopted originally perhaps out of a delicate consideration for the feelings of the patient, who always feels as if a mountain weight were taken from him, when the medical adviser, in whom he has confidence, pronounces after an examination, *It is only Bronchitis*.

I have thus been at some pains to describe what Bronchitis truly is, and what the meaning attached to the word in ordinary conversation, as I am satisfied that hitherto the term has not conveyed to common minds any clear, definite, distinct impression, but rather something ill-defined, mysterious, and obscure.

WHAT IS CLERGYMAN'S SORE THROAT?

It is the name which the common people have given to those symptoms which physicians call *Chronic Laryngitis*, and for shortness the single word " Laryngitis " is used.

Laryngitis is inflammation of the inner lining or mucous membrane of the Larynx, or voice making organs, which are situated at the top of the windpipe, forming outside the prominence known by the name of " Adam's Apple."

The symptoms of Laryngitis are a greater or less impairment of the voice, which is more or less hoarse, hollow, husky, cracked, irregular, uncontrolable, or weak. Some speak above a whisper only by a decided effort; others cannot speak above a whisper at all, for days, months, years; sometimes there is pain, and sometimes not; some complain of a pricking sensation if they sing, or swallow, or turn the neck quickly ; some have a cough, others none whatever; on almost all persons it has a wonderfully depressing influence, both on mind and body.   The great, the universal, the essential distinguishing symptom of Chronic Laryngitis, or Clergyman's Sore Throat, is a greater or less alteration of the voice, continuing for weeks or more at a time, and is often accompanied by an uneasy or painful feeling running up the sides of the neck towards the ears, or a heavy, dull aching about the region of Adam's Apple.

Clergymen's Sore Throat Ail, Laryngitis, Chronic Laryngitis, and what is often termed Bronchitis, (pronounced *Bron-kee-tis*) are one and the same disease, and will be called in these pages Laryngitis, (pronounced *Lare-in-gee-tis*,) it being the most scientific, appropriate, and expressive of all the terms used.

LARYNGITIS.

Laryngitis is a disease of the voice making organs, situated in the uppermost part of the windpipe, in the region of "Adams' apple," properly called *Thyroid cartilage.*

TRACHEITIS OR CROUP,

Is a disease of that portion of the windpipe, between the Thyroid cartilage and the little depression at the bottom of the neck, in front, just at the top of the breast bone.

BRONCHITIS,

Is a disease of the branches of the windpipe, below the depression above named. Simple bronchitis is what is usually called common cold, catarrh, &c.

CONSUMPTION,

Is a disease of the little air cells, or bladders, at the end of the branches of the windpipe.

BRONCHITIS, LARYNGITIS AND CONSUMPTION,

Are diseases widely different in their nature, locality, symptoms and modes of treatment.

I am not able, at this time, to think of any other three ailments whose methods of cure are so essentially different.

There are no three affections in the whole catalogue of human maladies, so often confounded, and taken, and treated one for another; hence the ill success which has so uniformly attended their management.

Bronchitis, needs internal remedies.
Laryngitis, requires washes to the parts, gargles and insufflations.
Consumption itself, calls for none of these things.

Bronchithis, is caused by the application of cold in some way, and in no other.

Laryngitis, is more often the result of accidental and temporary causes, such as indigestion, over exertion of the voice, suppressions, and the like.

Consumption, is generally inherited, and it is sufficient for one of the parents to have had a weakly, diseased constitution.

I never knew a case of Bronchitis, which was not attended with cough and large, weakening expectoration.

Laryngitis, is characterized by inconvenience, if not pain, in swallowing, hoarseness or huskiness, without cough necessarily at first, or much expectoration.

Consumption sometimes gives none of these symptoms; not even cough or expectoration, until within a few weeks of death.

In Bronchitis, the prominent symptoms are fullness and stricture, or tightness, binding in the breast, a "stopping up of the head," and watering of the nose and eyes.

In Laryngitis, the uniform symptom is a greater or less impairment of the voice, or some unnatural, troublesome feeling about the "swallow," especially in the act of swallowing.

In Consumption, there is the dry cough, the weakness, pain in the chest, shortness of breath in walking up hill, or ascending a pair of stairs, quick pulse and general falling away.

Consumption, is at one end of the breathing organs; Laryngitis, at the other; while Bronchitis is located between the two.

In Consumption, the slightest amelioration of the symptoms is seized upon with avidity.

In Throat diseases, evident improvement is looked upon doubtingly.

In Consumption, the spirits are cheerful; the patient is full of hope; is ever ready to embark in the occupations of life; and to every inquiry replies, "I'm better."

In Throat complaints, a man is dull, desponding, and listless; if he sits down, he is never ready to get up; but will lounge, and loaf, and mope about the house for hours together; it requires an effort to put one foot before another sometimes; and often he feels as if he would be happy were he sure that he never would have anything more to do as long as he lived.

While these striking differences exist in the three affections under consideration, it is at the same time true, that if allowed to go on unarrested; if permitted simply to "take their course;" if they are just "let alone," they do, with great uniformity, terminate in the same fatal symptoms.

We now see, that *Bronchitis, Clergyman's Sore Throat* and *Consumption*, are three different and distinct diseases; all connected with the breathing organs, yet different in their locality, in their causes, in their symptoms, and as will be seen, equally different in their treatment and mode of cure.

In order however to leave a clearer and more definite and lasting impression as to the nature, character causes, symptoms and cure of these three diseases, I will give a more particular description of their locality.

The top, or beginning, or entrance of the wind-pipe, is at the backpart, or root of the tongue; and behind that and nearer the neck bone, is the passage or canal, along which the food and drink pass to the stomach. Every particle of food which we swallow, passes directly over the top of the wind-pipe; and if a single atom "goes the wrong way," that is, goes into the wind-pipe instead of down the throat, all are familiar with what a tickling, hasty, dry cough it produces, followed by a great deal of hemming. But as the top of the wind-pipe never, perhaps, closes inself, (for if it did, no air could enter or escape from the lungs, and there would be suffocation,) how does it happen that the food and drink does not go down the first opening it comes to? The answer is, simply because just on the front edge of this opening, there is a little gristly substance, which stands erect (in its natural position) and works like a hinge; it is instantly affected by anything going from the mouth downwards, and instinctively closes hermetically—almost air-tight, perhaps quite so; and no sooner has it passed, than this little watchman stands erect again;

and, to personify, if he slept a moment, from the cradle to the grave, either while standing up or lying down, that moment we would cease to live; or if we lived at all, it would be with struggles most terrific—with grasping hands, agonized countenance, and blood-shot eye-balls. But here, happily for us, a watchman of our Maker's appointing, whether it be an atom or an angel, never fails of his duty—man only, the object of all these guardianships, comes short of it!! This little hinge is called *epiglottis*, because it shuts upon and closes the glottis, or top of the wind-pipe.

At the upper end of the wind-pipe, in a space of less that two inches in length, is the *Larynx*, which contains four muscles or strings, two or each side, one above the another, and less than half an inch apart, these are called *vocal chords* because they form and regulate the voice. The *Larynx* is subject to inflammation, like every other part of the body, producing, according to Dr. Stokes, no less than thirty-one different forms of disease! The general name for inflamed larynx, is *Laryngitis*, called *Clergyman's Sore Throat*, from the fact that so many clergymen of late years have been subject to it—not that they only are its victims; but as it impairs the voice, and hinders them in the exercise of their vocation, more attention is excited, than if scores of private individuals had it.

Next below the larynx; that is, the continuation of the laryngeal cylinder, is the trachea, or wind-pipe proper, beginning just below Adam's apple. When this is inflamed, it is called Tracheitis, (pronounced *Tra-kee-tis*,) known generally by the more familiar name of Croup, such as little children are frequently subject to in the spring and fall, and which they frequently die of.

The wind-pipe continues until it reaches the bottom of the neck, or top of the breast bone, where it divides into five branches, and dives down into the lungs, as a tree or bush branches out, "turned upside down." Two of these branches go to the left side of the breast, and three to the right; there, however, they divide off rapidly, until they become so minute as to be invisible. The branches are called Bronchi, or Bronchial tubes, and when inflamed, constitute the disease called Bronchitis.—See Plate.

But the extreme ends of these branches terminate in little bulbs or bladders; two, ten, or a dozen or more at each extremity, just as a branch or bush terminates in several leaves or buds, or berries, each one of which is larger in diameter than the extreme end of the branch from which it originates; these little bulbs or bladders are "roundish," and of all sizes, from a pin-head down to invisibility, and these are the lungs themselves to which the air is brought through the larynx, wind-pipe and bronchial tubes.

These little bladders, or vesicles, swell when the air comes in, and close in, when the air goes out, and it is this coming in and going out of the air that is the essence of life, that keeps the human machine in its ceaseless operations. When these little vesicles are inflamed, it is properly called *Pneumonitis;* and when this inflamation continues for a length of time, or their little blood vessels become so full that the contents exude out as it were, in little drops, which harden and become tubercles, and in time become yellow and rot away—*this is Consumption!*

It will be thus seen that:

CLERGYMAN'S SORE THROAT,	CROUP,	COMMON COLD,	CONSUMPTION
OR LARYNGITIS,	TRACHEITIS,	BRONCHITIS,	AND PHTHISIS,

Are inflammations of different parts of the same apparatus, to-wit: The tube which conveys the air from without, to the lungs: by keeping this in view, the reader will have hereafter a distinct and easy appreciation of the meaning of these terms.

Those who desire a more minute detail of the nature, form, functions, uses and diseases of the breathing organs, are referred to standard works which treat professedly of these things. What I most desire to communicate, is a knowledge of the nature, causes and symptoms of the diseases in question, so that if not affected, the people may avoid the cause; and if unfortunately, they are diseased, they may at once know it, and apply promptly for a remedy, before the malady has progressed to an incurable stage.

It may still further aid the general reader in forming a definite and correct idea of the different diseases of the throat and lungs, by considering the distinctive characteristics of the maladies under consideration, in the following parallels—

In Laryngitis, or Clergyman's Sore Throat.	In Tracheitis, or Croup.	In Bronchitis, or Common Cold.	In Pneumonitis, or Consumption.
The speech making organs are inflamed. Hence the voice is always more or less affected.	The wind-pipe is mainly inflamed, hence the breathing is more or less affected.	The Bronchial tubes are inflamed, hence a fullness in the breast, or stopping up, and a running from the nose and eyes.	The lungs themselves are inflamed, hence an impairment of all the powers of life.
The voice is always altered; affects adults mainly.	The breathing is always obstructed, and affects children mainly.	There is cough, and running at the nose and eyes; affects all ages and classes.	Always a wasting of the Lungs, and none are totally exempt.
Disinctive symptom: a chronic impairment of the voice.	Distinctive symptom: a kind of barking cough.	Distinctive symptom: Fullness of head, breast, eyes and nose; stricture in the breast. and large expectoration.	Distinctive symptoms: a gradual wasting of the strength and flesh, with cough and quick pulse.

It will now be understood that Laryngitis or Clergyman's Sore Throat is a disease the situation of which is at the top or beginning of the wind-pipe, and that its proper symptom is an alteration of the voice.

That Bronchitis is a disease of the branches of the wind-pipe, and its characteristic symptom is more or less fullness and discharge from the nose, eyes, head and breast, with cough and expectoration.

That Consumption is a disease of the lungs themselves, which are situated at the extreme ends of the branches of the wind-pipe, and its great general feature is cough, wasting and death.

That Clergyman's Sore Throat and Consumption are situated at the extreme, and opposite ends of the breathing organs, and Bronchitis in the parts between the two.

That Clergyman's Sore Throat or Laryngitis is an altered voice.

That Consumption is a steady decay.

That Bronchitis is fullness, coughing, binding and discharge from the eyes, nose and head, and copious expectoration of that which is formed in the Bronchial passages.

I have personally known some of the most obstinate and incurable forms of Laryngitis to be attended with no other appreciable symptom than an altered voice; although in mild cases the voice is not perceptibly altered, but in its stead a frequent barking, hemming, &c.

There are cases of Consumption of the most fatal character, where no cough was ever noticed until within three weeks of death, but these were attended with great debility and wasting.

I never knew a case of Bronchitis not attended with cough, copious and varied expectoration and discharge, more or less from the nose and eyes.

A tree or bush pulled up, the roots being cut close off, and turned upside down, bears no unapt resemblance to the breathing apparatus in the natural position.

The Root,	Body,	Branches	Leaves answering to
The Larynx,	Wind-pipe,	Bronchial Tubes,	Air Cells or Lungs,

The Root being the seat of Clergyman's Sore Throat,
The body   "   of Common Croup,
The Branches,   "   of Bronchitis,
The Leaves.   "   of Consumption.

Perhaps the reader now thinks it extremely easy to tell whether he has Bronchitis, Laryngitis—or Consumption, but unfortunately new difficulties commence at this very point from the following causes.

Common custom has made these *three* diseases *two;* and acknowledges but two names, *Bronchitis* and *Consumption:* whatever cases get well are called "Bronchitis;" those that die. are called "Consumption."

Another great source of difficulty is that Bronchitis, Clergyman's Sore Throat and

Consumption, constantly mingle their Symptoms, run into one another, and produce one another; that is, Bronchitis may end in Clergyman's Sore Throat or Consumption.

Clergyman's Sore Throat very often, indeed, almost always ends in Consumption, while in many instances Laryngitis is a sequela of Consumption; and I have known cases where the symptoms of the whole three seemed to be concentrated in one unfortunate individual. In short, these diseases so mask one another, that the most eminent of living physicians have given various opinions of the same case, at the same time, and death has shown that all were mistaken. *See page ninety-nine of the fifth Edition*—REMARKABLE INSTANCES.

Another source of difficulty is that some other diseases occasionally give rise to the most marked symptoms of Consumption, so that veteran practitioners of a quarter of a century, have been entirely deceived. *See page ninety-eight, fifth Edition.*

If Bronchitis, Clergyman"s Sore Throat and Consumption are merged into the two names of *Bronchitis* and *Consumption;* if popular usage decrees that all who recover, have had *"only Bronchitis,"* and that only those who die, had Consumption; if too, these diseases constantly run into one another, constantly commingle their symptoms, and are masked by other diseases, totally different from them, and to such a degree that eminent men of long and large practice, have been utterly at fault or at a loss to discriminate—what is to be done? Is any remedy proposed? any remedy that can be relied upon, any remedy that has been fully tried and that stands the test of repetition and of time? In answer, I think the mode to be proposed in these pages, will enable me to say surely and truthfully of a given case "that man cannot have lost any portion of his lungs by disease;" or of another "his lungs are in a state of decay, he has lost the use of one third of them, and he is in the last stages of consumptive disease." This mode of examining the condition of the lungs, enables me to tell with certainty what proportion of a man's lungs are rendered useless to him by disease, even down to the two hundredth part of the whole; but if on the other hand a person comes up to certain relative physical requisitions, it is utterly impossible, whatever else may be the matter with him, that his lungs should be in a state of decay, disease, or even of mal-action. This is done on the principle suggested by Abernethy, that is, measuring the lungs themselves, in a manner so simple, so convincing, so satisfactory, so demonstrable, that it has afforded me the greatest pleasure to explain it to those who have called upon me. The general principle is this, if a man's lungs in perfect, healthful action hold so much air, say two hundred and fifty cubic inches on an average, it is easy to perceive that if half his lungs are gone, he can only hold half as much air. The details are too prolix for these pages, but five minutes are sufficient for a perfectly clear and convincing explanation to any one who may call for it in person, as one minute's sight of an object frequently gives a more perfect idea of it to the beholder, than a whole volume of plates and written descriptions.

In this way says the London Lancet, it is proven by actual experiment, that a man's lungs, found after death to have been tuberculated to the extent of one cubic inch, had been by that amount of tubercularization controlled in their action to the extent of more that forty inches. It is very apparent then, that this mode of examination detects the presence of tubercles in their earliest formation, which is in fact the only time to attack Consumption successfully and surely; and when attempted at the early stage, before it is at all fixed in the system, the certainty of success in warding off the danger, of curing the disease, is as great as that of warding off the cholera or perfectly curing it, if attempted at the first appearance of the premonitory symptoms, and as when cholera is present in a community, every person who has three or more passages from the bowels within twenty-four hours, ought to be considered as attacked with cholera, and should act accordingly, so when a man has tubercles in his lungs to the extent of impairing their functions for a dozen inches, that is when his lungs do not, with other symptoms, hold enough air by a dozen inches, he should consider himself as having consumption, and should act accordingly and with the assurance that in four cases out of five, human life would be saved by it. And as thousands have died with cholera by hoping they did not have it, or denying they had it, although warned by the usual symptoms of its commencement, until its existence was so apparent to the commonest observer as to render a hope of cure impossible, so precisely is it in consumption, people will not take warning of the symptoms in their own persons, which have in thousands of others terminated in certain death, but go on day after day without reason, hoping that the symptoms will go away of themselves, and steadily deny that they have the disease, until remedy is hopeless.

I have already said, that when Consumption has once fixed itself in the system, recovery is not probable; but if the disease is not fixed, and is only in its commencement, it may be certainly distinguished in its early stage, by the new means which I have advocated; and in very many instances averted; not so much by "taking things," as by letting them alone: not by confining the natural motion of the limbs by braces and supporters, but by allowing them the freest possible action: not by the application of Blisters and Plasters, which only interfere with the natural action of the skin, but by exciting and promoting that natural action: not by administering expectorants, which only weaken the system by hastening its drains, and producing nausea, but by regulating and controlling these drains, the expectoration being loosened by nature's means, when desirable. In consumption, I give nothing to purge, or which can by any possibility have a weakening effect; I give no artificial stimulant, which requires to be increased in frequency or quantity, or loses its effect altogether, or at last requires so much as to injure the tone of the stomach by preventing it from deriving proper nourishment from the food, and the patient rapidly sinks into the grave after having given a glowing certificate, or told dozens of people what a wonderful effect the Syrup was having in his case. This is the true history of all the "Syrups," "Cough Mixtures," and "Wild Cherry Balsams," sold in the shops for coughs, cold and consumption; and without doubt the reader can easily recollect cases among his neighbors, such as I have detailed.

I give no medicine to increase the expectoration, because the lungs are already expectorated away too fast. I give no medicine to remove the cough or smother it, for cough is the agent which nature sends to remove accumulations from the lungs, otherwise they would fill up and the patient would suffocate. I do not confine a patient in-doors, but keep him out as much as possible. I do not send them to a warm climate, if sent they must be, but to a colder and more bracing one—to a more condensed and purer atmosphere. I do not counsel them to leave the facilities and comforts and attention of home, to pine away in some distant country tavern, or pig-sty boarding house, or icicled fashionable hotel—these are not the places for a body worn away by disease, and wasted by long nights of incessant cough or drenching night sweats, cold and clammy as the grave; nor for a mind made timid by constant pain, and weakened by its own incessant and restless workings. If any man in the wide world needs them, it is the consumptive, who should have around him every comfort, every convenience, every facility which unbounded wealth or undying affection can procure. The light step, the soft whisper, the affectionate inquiry, the cheerful voice, the friendly smile, the tireless watching, and the sleepless eye—all these, and a thousand other nameless attentions, he needs, and needs them every day and every hour. To leave home for any length of time is a piece of advice which ought never to be given in a case of decided consumption; it is not applicable in any stage of actual consumptive disease, and an observant practitioner will never give it. Voyages at sea, and locations on the seashore or lake coasts, are unsuitable, pernicious, and deadly in their ultimate effects. The reasons for these opinions, which will be considered unusual at least by many readers, may be seen at length at page 106, 5th ed. of my book.

I wish it could be as deeply felt as it is strictly true, throughout this broad continent, in every mansion of its merchant princes, and in every fisherman's hut and squatter's cabin, that the permanent arrest of consumptive disease in its latter stages and its effectual eradication when only in its first beginnings, is to be accomplished by one and the same system of means, and which no *internal medicine* hitherto known to man has ever yet been able to accomplish, nor does this system of means require any.

In the treatment of any case purely consumptive, two things only are needed, and they are needed always, and under all circumstances :

A greater consumption of pure fresh, condensed air.

A greater digestion of nutritious food.

A man must have more air for his lungs, and more flesh for his bones. A consumptive is always short of breath and deficient in flesh. No medicine can ever give air to the lungs, nor can it impart nutriment to the system. It is the pure air which the lungs receive which purifies the blood, and it is plain, substantial food introduced into the stomach which gives nutriment and strength and flesh to the system. My practice, therefore, in simple consumptive disease is, to force the lungs to consume a larger and larger quantity of *pure, fresh, condensed* air every day, and to cause the digestive apparatus to derive from the food a greater and greater amount of nutriment; hence, as my patients are getting well, they walk faster, run farther without fatigue, eat more food, digest it better, and consequently increase in flesh, and while this is going on, the cough, in all curable cases, gradually and spontaneously disappears, without doing anything for it; it disappears because it is eradicated, and not because it is smothered up by balsams, drops, syrups, and all the long catalogue of life-destroying poisons, which are sold under the name of patent medicines, by the unsuspecting in their credulity, or by the unprincipled in their wilful recklessness of human life.

One of the greatest difficulties in the successful treatment of Consumption is, that the stomach and bowels are deranged; the appetite may be moderately good, and the bowels for the most part regular, yet for all that, they are not in a condition sufficiently healthful to impart to the system the nutriment which the food contains, but which they are not able to eliminate; hence, the universal complaint, *what I eat does not seem to strengthen me any;* but this very condition is always and inevitably aggravated by every dose of patent medicine swallowed for coughs and the like; because every one of them, without any exception, as every respectable physician knows, and every honest, intelligent druggist will acknowledge, has more or less opium in some form or other, and this is impossible to be taken, even a single time, without having a tendency to make the liver torpid, to derange the stomach, and to constipate the bowels.

I do not wish it to be understood that I give no internal medicine under any circumstances, nor that I undervalue its remedial efficacy. I have only said that a man does not need internal medicine when he has simple, uncomplicated Consumption. The majority of persons who come to me have other ailments in addition to the breast or throat complaint; some have piles, others dyspepsia, liver complaint, neuralgia, whites, falling of the womb, heart-burns, "fainty spells," pains about the shoulders, spitting of blood, and the like. When that is the case, I am obliged to cure these things first, before I can proceed a single step towards eradicating the consumptive disease; and to do these things I must use the medicines which educated and experienced practitioners usually employ.

How I give pure, fresh, condensed air to the lungs to purify the blood, and how I give increased nutriment to the system, to strengthen it by enriching the blood, I have neither the room nor the disposition to tell in these pages, because they are not written to instruct medical men in the cure of disease, but to instruct the common people, that they may understand thoroughly what are the symptoms of diseases of the throat and lungs at an early stage, and may feel the importance of making immediate application for their total eradication while such a thing is possible.

The best physicians in the land, with the experience and skill of a quarter of a century, but too often fail to conduct a case of common consumption of the lungs to a favorable and successful termination, and no one of any intelligence could expect to have the requisite knowledge communicated to him in the few pages of a shilling pamphlet; and I must say that the man who could be tempted to tinker with his constitution, from any knowledge that he could gain from any source in half a day, or a much longer period, when he would not be willing, with equal facilities of instruction, to attempt the mending of an old shoe, such a man does not deserve a constitution. Still, in the *Appendix Edition* of this publication, I have given the treatment in some of the more remarkably successful cases under my care. It is simply an addition to this publication; and not supposing that a large issue would be sold, I have published but a few copies. Any person sending me a dollar, free of postage, to New Orleans after November 1st, or to Cincinnati after the 15th of May of each year, will have a paper covered copy sent by mail, or a full bound one if sent for by private hand. This Appendix Edition will also contain the letters of persons applying to me from a distance, describing their own cases and their successful termination, and that too without my ever having seen them. These may be peculiarly interesting to many, as showing how persons may be cured of serious and complicated maladies of long standing, simply by sending them printed and written directions from time to time.

CAUSES OF THROAT AFFECTIONS.

Of that form of Laryngitis which I am denominating *Clergymen's Sore Throat*, it is sufficient for practical purposes to say, that it is any increasing impairment in the voice for several weeks in duration. This alteration of the voice may arise from an inflammation of the larynx, caused by indigestion, diseased liver, suppressed evacuations, too sudden healing of old sores, too hasty driving in of any breaking out of the skin, whether that breaking out be called measles, tetter, erysipelas, scarlet fever, rash, itch, or anything else that can be named; it may be caused by venereal ulcers, by sudden checking of perspiration, by keeping the feet damp for several hours, by sitting on cold stones or damp seats for some time; by speaking too loud; by singing or teaching too much; by excessive exercise and fatigue in a warm and crowded room, and then going out suddenly into the cold air, especially in damp, raw, windy weather; by sleeping in a position where the wind blows on the sleeper, even in summer; by going from a very cold atmosphere into a heated apartment; by breathing the steam of boiling water; by inhaling poisonous vapors, or the loaded atmosphere of cabinet or carpenter shops, stone cutters, gold beaters, iron, brass, or steel filers, and the like; cotton factories; the close apartments in which steam engines are usually worked, and such like places; by the excessive use of mercury; by demoralizing indulgences in secret; by habitual intemperance, whether the person be ever actually drunk or not; by a hereditary taint; by a scrofulous or tuberculous constitution—the slightest causes are sufficient to bring it on in these three last named cases; by common colds, frequently repeated; swollen tonsils. It matters not by which of all these causes the voice is impaired, immediate attention should be given to it, the cause sought out, the proper appliances made, and the disease averted.

The causes of Clergymen's Sore Throat are all such as are capable of producing inflammations when applied to mucous surfaces in any part of the body, for example: A common cold, frequently repeated, especially in persons accustomed to use spirituous liquors, such persons being always more subject to disease, and when attacked, suffer more, and are by far less apt to recover than those who never taste spirits, beers, ciders, or any such things.

EXCESSIVE EXERTIONS OF THE VOICE—A CASE.

A clergyman and his companion amused themselves one day in the woods by experimenting which could speak the loudest. The minister was the victor, but experienced a sharp pricking sensation in the throat, yet took no special notice of it: next morning, however, it was worse; he became hoarse, had a troublesome hacking cough, followed by weakness, emaciation, and night sweats. His friends gave him up as lost. He was obliged to abandon the ministry for three years and a half; but he got well and hearty, and can speak in public three times on the Sabbath with ease, and has been doing it for years.

Moderate speaking, if in crowded rooms during winter. Clergymen, Congress_ men, and Legislators are subject to these causes:

A CASE.

A member of the Legislature called on me and made this statement: "You see I am a square-built man, with a well developed chest. For eighteen years I had the most perfect health, having pursued an active, out-door business life. I was sent to the Legislature. It was an exciting session. The Chamber was often crowded to excess; the air became heated and foul, while there were cold, piercing, damp winds without. I spoke occasionally. In two months my appetite was gone; with a harrassing cough through the day, with expectoration, high fevers every afternoon, red cheeks; in four months more, I became what you see me now, I am weak, without energy, have drenching night sweats, and have lost forty pounds of flesh."

I told this gentleman that there was a high degree of inflamation in the throat, that it was extending rapidly to the lungs, and would then be without remedy. Such was the case, for he died within three months.

Wounds, blows, contusions, fish bones, cherry stones, tacks, &c., lodging in the larynx, are common cause of throat affections.

A CASE.

A man came to me who had the sore throat from having, some time before, swallowed a copper tack, bent at the sharp ead like a fish hook—making an ulcer. Dry tongue, a very bad taste in the mouth, a feeling of binding and heaviness along the front of the breast and across it, constant for several months just preceding, and an almost ceaseless gnawing at the stomach, for the last few months, keeping his bowels constantly disordered, with a difficulty of breathing, constantly growing worse, especially on exercise; "expectorate a great deal every day, half a gill, of the worst kind of stuff, bloody, stringy, and bubbly." Within two months he ceased to come to my office, "for nothing was the matter," as he expressed himself to me. The tack had lodged in the wind-pipe.

N. B.—I will here mention, not a cause, but a frequent accompaniment of sore throat, which those interested will do well to remember. Persons will complain, not of a sore throat, but of a gnawing, or other bad feeling, at the pit of the stomach, sometimes a swelling, an instinctive disposition to pull the clothing from the stomach with the fingers, as if it would give relief to loosen them, and when describing their case, they point to the upper part of the breast in front, as a source of uneasy feeling. The cause of this uneasy feeling in the breast may be, that from the diseased state of the larynx, the air has not a naturally free passage to and from the lungs—while the difficulty in the stomach may be produced by ulcers about the top of the larynx, which constantly generate a foul sanies, or "ugly matter," which, every time a person swallows, is carried down into the stomach; enough in thought at least, to produce the worst kind of dispepsia, and undermine the strongest constitution in a few months. Persons have come to me with a mass of foul ulcers in the throat, and "did not know anything was the matter." It is because they are too far down to be seen, without proper instruments are applied.

EXTENSION OF OTHER DISEASES TO THE THROAT.

Ulcers and sores of various kinds, being the extension of other diseases, are removed with admirable promptness and certainty, when proper applications are made to the spots affected—the same may be said of ulcers that are causing the patient to speak through the nose,"—these are also arrested and cured at once. Throat disease is not unfrequently brought on by causes so unseen, working out the death in so insidious a manner, with a progress so gradual and so slow, that its advance is undreamed of, until some sudden symptom wakes up the patient and the patient's physician to a proper sense of the impending danger.

HOW AM I TO KNOW WHETHER I HAVE THE DISEASE OR NOT?

When a person reads that there are so many causes of this disease, to several of which he knows himself to have been exposed; that it is so much like consumption, in many instances laying the foundation of it—that it sometimes destroys life in a few days; that in others it insinuates itself into the system to an almost fatal extent, without the patient knowing anything about it; and when it is present, making death possible any hour, from the ulcer eating into the gullet or other adjacencies; from the swelling and closure of the vocal chords at midnight, causing instant death; when these things are taken into consideration, the above question becomes one of absorbing interest, especially to one who has any slight uneasiness about the throat, of some weeks standing.

I do not at present remember one single disease, whose early stage is infallibly indicated by any one symptom; but any alteration of the voice, or any pain in swallowing, or on pressing the throat about the wind-pipe, should excite an anxious inquiry; and the anxiety should be increased in proportion as are observed uneasiness about the top of the breast bone; frequent indescribable taste in the mouth; "ugly" expectoration; a feeling as if you wanted to get something out of the back of the mouth; a sticky, clammy, or tough, stringy feeling there; a frequent bringing up of something with a single hawk, or clearing the throat, without coughing; or a disposition to swallow frequently, as if you felt you could get rid of it by swallowing, and yet fail to do so—but if there is pain on pressing about Adam's apple to one side or the other; or if you do not swallow without some soreness or twinge, or pricking sensation, or if in swallowing liquids, they turn through the nostrils, you may be sure of it!!

Laryngitis, or *Clergymen's Sore Throat,* sometimes begins very insidiously as a common cough, with hoarseness, the cough not attracting particular attention, until it has lasted for a considerable length of time, and seriously injured the general health, with the tissues of the part affected. The most marked symptoms are a husky, dry cough, with—

Soreness or pain in the region of Adam's apple, felt sometimes on pressure, sometimes in the act of swallowing, as if a fish bone were sticking there.

The most constant sign is the change of voice, which varies much in degree and kind, while there is not the slightest cough whatever.

There is a peculiarity in the hoarseness, which is of a deep, a loose or mucous kind, or it is dry or squeaking or wheezing hoarseness, accompanied by an occasional cough, with a fine, sometimes almost indistinct whistling noise.

A *sudden* loss of voice may occur in consequence of slight disease of some of the ligaments, or a nervous affection of the muscles, and may not be permanent, but where a voice becomes gradually more and more cracked until it is at last lost, there is progressive destruction of the vocal apparatus, for which there is no remedy.

In some cases the defect of the voice is only perceptible on speaking loud, or in any attempt to vary the tone, for the patient instinctively acquires a habit of speaking in that tone and degree in which the voice is best produced. In perhaps half the cases of Laryngitis, there is no pain until the disease is very far advanced, there is, however, an increased tenderness in the part, so that breathing cold air, or any hurry of the circulation, readily excites a short hacking cough; as it advances, the cough is loose and continuous.

When there is an offensive expectoration, it relieves the breathing more or less, although the voice may suffer more, and there may be more pain and soreness in coughing; this indicates the presence of an ulcer. The breathing, sooner or later, becomes affected, coming on mostly at night, and on over exertion.

Sometimes the attacks of difficult breathing becomes so severe that the patient is left exhausted. At other times he is prevented from lying down; and in the interval, the hissing sound of the breathing indicates some degree of permanent impediment to the air.

In many instances, the throat affection is accompanied by progressive emaciation, hectic fever, night sweats, and other signs of Consumption of the lungs, and the patient is ultimately worn down by cough and weakness, and is perhaps carried off by diarrhœa.

GENERAL HISTORY OF THROAT AIL.

The general history of the beginning, progress, and end of a case of Laryngitis, is as follows:

An uneasy feeling is present in the upper part of the throat, causing a frequent tendency to swallow, as if some obstruction might be removed thereby. In other cases, there is a constant hemming or hawking, in order to clear the throat of some sticky or glutinous stuff, adhering to the back part of it; then, the voice is not of that clear, ringing sound as formerly; or if it is made clear, it requires an effort, which shows that something is wrong; for nature works without an effort; after a while the effort becomes such as to cause fatigue. The voice has to be pushed out as it were; at length it becomes hoarse or cracked, after unusual speaking or reading; this is more perceptible after meals, or towards evening; some soreness begins now to be felt in the region of Adam's apple. There may be, as yet, no cough; and for weeks and months, and even years, except occasionally, it makes no perceptible progress, even getting better; but becomes worse again from exposure to changes of weather, and other causes; and thus it alternates, until the patient becomes exhausted in his efforts to get rid of it; the strength declines; the cough appears; the constitution yields, and death closes the scene.

It must be remembered that, sometimes, no cough makes its appearance until within a few weeks of death, but the voice becomes more and more cracked, discordant and husky; it requires the utmost effort to enounce a word above a whisper; the whole body seems to exert itself in the pronunciation of every syllable and not only the throat, but the whole system is wearied with the effort; but always unattended with extreme pain, in or about the throat. Sometimes the voice becomes utterly extinct previous to dissolution.

In the progress of the disease, ulcers form in the throat, so far down as not to be visible to the common eye, and these ulcers pour out, day by day, enormous quantities of the most offensive stuff, matter, blood, mucus, pure or mixed, a great deal of which is got rid of by expectoration, a whole pint of it in a day sometimes; another part goes by way of the stomach, and people wonder "where so much corruption comes from!" and assure the physician that they "must have spit up all the lungs before now;" and yet, on a proper examination, the lungs will be found unbroken and undecayed. While this affords encouragement to persons who appear to have Consumption, to have their cases properly examined, perchance the lungs may happily be sound, notwithstanding the threatening nature of appearances; it at the same time points out the necessity of prompt attention in all cases where there is any ailment about the throat, or any alteration of the voice whatever.

Many distinguished names, such as Piorry, Chomel, Louis, Belloc, Andral, Columbat De L'Isere, Sir Charles Bell, Stokes, Green, and others, bear the most unhesitating testimony to this important and interesting truth: "There can be no doubt that a person may have all the apparent signs of Consumption of the Lungs, in cousequence of the throat affection, and the lungs themselves be free from disease."

In view of this, how strongly does the irresistible conviction fasten itself upon the mind of every reflecting reader, that many have been hastily abandoned, as being in the last stages of consumption, because they had cough, emaciation, night sweats, and difficult breathing, when a skilful physician would have detected in the throat alone, a sufficient cause for these alarming symptoms, and, by a short course of judicious treatment, have rescued them from an untimely grave.

A talented and distinguished preacher called upon me, in New Orleans last winter, for an examination and opinion of his case. His friends had supposed his to be a case of hopeless consumption. I considered it one of throat disease in the main, and treated it accordingly. In two months he writes to me:—

"Dear Sir: Your prescriptions began in a few days to act like a charm. My cough is more than half abated—digestion improved fifty per cent., strength and spirits in like proportion—nothing seemed against me but too frequent pulse, my throat and voice improved wonderfully, and my respiration very much helped," &c.

The rapid and thorough improvement in this case could only have taken place on the ground of my opinion being correct as to the character of his ailment—and yet he had been sent an interminable journey south, from Kentucky through Florida, and, as he informed me, he "got worse all the time." What a world of distress and anxiety, and what a large expenditure of time and money might have been saved to this gentleman, had a more truthful opinion been formed of his case before he left home.

Another clergyman, after having been under treatment for some time, writes me, and after relating the favorable changes which had taken place, says: "And, permit me to say, Doctor, that I shall ever cherish, with grateful remembrance, the day I first visited your office for advice and prescription, and that you may long live to relieve the sufferings of the human family, and enjoy that happiness which a consciousness of doing good gives its possessor, is the prayer of your obedient servant." '

A FATAL CASE.

There are sometimes persons who cannot understand how it is that they can be in a very dangerous condition, when they can eat and drink and walk about the streets, and have no pain or soreness except some hoarseness, or a little pricking or twinging in the throat on pressure, or on swallowing, or on a sudden turn of the

B

head, or other movement of the body. A case: a gentleman of some distinction, of polished manners, and whose life was of considerable importance to the community, called at my office wishing to know my opinion of his case. On a careful examination, I told him he was suffering more from a throat disease than anything else, and that there was no efficient remedy. As I could do him no material good, I dismissed him, expecting to see him no more. Early next morning he returned, and said, "you must do something for my throat." I prescribed, and he got better rapidly, very rapidly. Knowing, however, that he could not recover, and seeing that every day he was cherishing new hopes of life, I thought it best to acquaint his wife, to whom he had not long been married, that I considered him in a dangerous condition, and advised an immediate return to his friends, assuring her, at the same time, in the most positive terms, that he was liable to die within any hour. He could not be induced to assent to my views, and I advised him to call in another physician. He did so, and I withdrew. Within ten days, though apparently better, his wife heard a singular noise while her husband was sleeping, and before she could go to the family apartment to give the alarm and return, he was dead. This sudden death sometimes arises from ulcers forming in the windpipe or its branches, and closing up the passages so that no air can pass; or an ulcer bursts and fills up the passages with matter, so as to suffocate. Sometimes the ulcers eat through the sides of the air passages, and making communications with adjoining parts, produce irritation, inflammation and death.

A gentleman called at my office with a distressing hoarseness of voice, but no soreness, it required a great effort for him to speak distinctly. He had just placed himself under the care of a physician, who was said to have hand some success in curing throat diseases; but hearing that I was in town, he called on me to know what I thought of his condition. I was obliged to say that he would die in a few days, and declined prescribing; first, because I knew that I could do him no material good; and, second, I considered it would not be just toward his physician to abandon his treatment without giving it a fair trial. I saw him on the street several times afterwards, but within ten days I was hastily summoned to see him, and found him dead from suffocation.

It ought to be extensively known that there are several forms of throat disease, which render those who have them liable to sudden death; this is especially true of acute and chronic Laryngitis, from swelling, inflammation, or exudation about the upper part of the Larynx, which close the sides, and prevent breathing. This is very liable to come on in the night, during sleep; the breath is gradually stopped, the person becomes unconscious; instinctive struggles may give the alarm, but death usually ensues, before any person can be called; of this Washington died.

This sudden death may occur at any time to those who have enlarged Tonsils. When enlarged, they ought to be taken out at once, unless judicious and safe means are used by an intelligent physician, to cause the swelling to subside. For if treated injudiciously, they become hardened, and are liable to a cancerous affection, which is perhaps the most terribly painful of all diseases, as well as fatal. Persons should be careful how they employ gargles and washes, and refuse to use them un_ less recommended by a respectable physician.

CAUSES AND CASES FROM TROUSSEAU AND OTHERS.

C. M. noticed that public speaking was followed by some soreness in the throat, which usually wore off in a day or two; in a year or two it was painful to make a speech, and he was compelled to desist altogether from making public addresses. In time, every attempt to speak a word required an effort which was followed by weari_ ness; there is a constant disposition to swallow or clear the throat, increased by talking or catching cold—appetite good—sleep sound—general health uninjured. If there is several days rest, he begins to feel well, but if any attempt is made to speak for fifteen minutes, the soreness in the throat returns.

A woman, while sitting on a stone bench in February, was attacked with sudden hoarseness, this continued, grew worse until the voice was lost altogether; a little pain in the throat, shortness of breath on the least exercise; was three months getting well.

Mrs. P. took cold by being exposed in the Park in Versailles, in August, followed by a hoarseness which nothing could control. In two years her voice was altogether extinct. In two months more there was oppression and shortness of breath if she walk▪ fast; in two weeks more this oppression became constant during the night, often threatening suffocation; and death took place in two years and a half from the first hoarseness.

A tall man, strong constitution, good figure, aged thirty-three, had hoarseness every winter for five years, then there was cough, irregular chills, clear expectoration, very sensitive to cold, copious night sweats, daily fever, voice then changed some, throat became painful, then drinks began to return by the nose, appetite bad, digestion imperfect, casting up after meals, gradual falling away, heat in the throat, loss of voice, thick greenish expectoration, diarrhœa and death.

A man thirty years old, delicate, subject to frequent colds for eighteen months past; with pains in the throat and hoarseness; voice hoarse and broken; expectoration thick and tough; often put his hands to his throat as if there were some obstruction there; had fits of coughing which were stifling, this grew painfully severe; and finally died of suffocation.

A gentleman aged forty-two was attacked in the street one morning in August, with a fit of suffocation; he could not proceed; a dry rough hoarse cough came on, with shortness of breath. In two weeks had another attack and died.

A vigorous Dutch courier was subject to cold every winter for eight years, but last winter it was worse, with sore throat, and obstinate hoarseness; emaciated very rapidly, with complete loss of voice; acute pain in the throat when he swallows either liquid or solid food; a tender spot on the side of Adam's apple when pressed with the finger; expectoration streaked with yellow at times, at others it is viscid, small. opaque, and swimming in a sort of mucilage; night sweats on face and chest; general debility and death.

A gentleman, aged fifty, had an eruption over the body; it disappeared, but a pain in the throat ca▪▪▪▪▪immediately, with a feeling of oppression; expectoration smelt badly. I▪▪▪▪▪two there was a cough, hoarse voice, with a tough, sticky expectoration;▪▪▪▪▪in the throat, especially on swallowing—and even of liquids; fallin▪▪▪▪of voice and death.

A large, spare▪▪▪▪▪ty-two, a porter, noticed his voice changing for thirteen months, becoming h▪▪▪for the last six weeks, until the voice was almost lost; difficult breathing, painful swallowing; wakes in starts from sleep, and died of suffocation.

B. W. felt uneasy about the throat frequently, inclining him to swallow or to clear the throat, as something appeared to be sticking there ; now and then there was a little hoarseness, especially towards evening, or after speaking or reading ; occasional dryness in the throat ; some burning feeling at the side of the neck ; unnatural sensation at top of breast-bone ; sometimes a feeling of tightness there ; in the course of the year he found it required some little effort when after silence he began to talk, a kind of instinctive summoning of strength about the breast, in order to enable him to speak clearly and distinctly ; after awhile, whenever spoken to, he would be compelled to give a hem or two before attempting to reply, as if conscious that something must be cleared away first.

Several cases of this last kind, especially in young men, were entirely cured without a further expense than the first week's prescriptions.

A clergyman says: " I had spoken a great deal for six weeks, which left some hoarseness, otherwise quite well. Soon the hoarseness was such as to reduce me to a whisper if I conversed only a few minutes ; the throat inside looked very red, with large blotches or hillocks on the back part of it, and a slimy stuff was always colleeting there, and when I would hawk it away, there would sometimes be streaks of blood in it ; occasionally a little pain there. I quit preaching, and kept the house for several months, and nothing does me any good."

None of these cases came under my care ; they are given to show how often a permanent hoarseness or huskiness, or loss of voice; or soreness in the throat, or painful pricking sensation in swallowing; or a gradual change of voice, end in death, sooner or later, if neglected; and the hope is, that the reader will take warning by these, and by timely application, save himself from a death at once painful and often extremely sudden, coming on in the dead hour of night, when there is no unusual or alarming symptom the preceding day.

LOSS OF VOICE.

On the 9th of March, a distinguished clergyman, young and of great promise, made to me the following statement : " Unusual circumstances compelled me to perform an immense amount of clerical labor, the work of three men; but it seemed unavoidable. I broke down, and was attacked seven months ago, in apparent health, with a sudden fit of coughing, which lasted three hours. I lost my voice ; went to New York for medical advice ; thence to Jamaica, in the West Indies ; returned to the United States, still an invalid, not having dared to preach since my first attack."

He had night and morning cough, and the usual auscultatory signs of the loss of the upper portion of one lung. He was spitting up daily, quantities of thick, heavy, yellow matter. He said he was engaged to be married to a lovely woman, but that if his was a hopeless case, he could not reconcile it to his conscience to marry. He had great personal popularity, and was almost idolized by his people, and a large circle of family connections. Here was a case well calculated to excite the highest interest of a physician.

On the 3d of April following, I find the following memorandum in my note-book: "Reports ' my voice and throat are as clear and well as they ever were_in my life,' and left for home." Some months afterwards he called upon me to say that he was preaching with his usual ease and comfort, and was married.

ANOTHER CASE.

On the 21st of July a gentleman came to see me, from Detroit—married, aged thirty-six—saying, " In November last, I was taken with hoarseness, which, in three or four weeks, was reduced to a whisper, and has continued about the same ever since. My general health is excellent; no cough, no pain, no ailment of any description, except an inability to speak louder than a whisper. I have tried every different practice—allopathy, hydropathy, homœopathy, and the botanic system, without the slightest advantage. My friends and physicians advised me to remain at home; that it was utterly useless to try anything else; and that it would be a waste of time and money to travel such a distance to see you."

It would have been very gratifying to have cured this case; but I have not done so, yet there is a prospect of his recovery. In one week after he came to me, he could speak a word or two at a time above a whisper; for ten days after that no other advance was made, and he began to be discouraged; the next day there was a farther improvement, and he urged me to use stronger remedies, and more frequently. But I never consult a patient's wishes or opinions. I allow those who come to me only one liberty—the liberty of ceasing their attendance at my office, the moment they think I am doing them no good—to stay only as long as they choose, and to come back whenever they are ready, or to stay away, as they think proper; so they get well, it is immaterial whether I cure them, or some other person does it. My earnest wish always is, that they may get well by some means or other. If a patient thinks he is not getting on fast enough, I would not blame him or get out of humor with him for trying some one else, for it is the very thing I would do myself if I were treated for a serious disease, and did not think I was getting better. If my health and life were threatened, I would try every body, and every thing that held out the least rational prospect of success, and would keep on trying until I came to the right place; and I do not blame others if they do the same thing. Those who may come to me, after reading this, will please bear it in mind. The patient of whom I was speaking, when this digression began, has now been with me about a month. He is able to sing some, and can speak several consecutive sentences in a loud voice, requiring however, some effort. He has not been confined to the house a single hour, and taken no medicine beyond a few pills, to remove costiveness; I have made no blisters, or running sores, and have given him no pain. I believe he will get well if he continues the treatment. If he does, it will be an additional triumph; if he does not get entirely well, it is no discouragement to me, for I do not expect to cure every case, and never have held out any such promise; men are not immortal, and all are born to die.

I designed the phrases *Throat Disease, Laryngitis, Clergyman's Sore Throat,* to include any affection of the Larynx, or the parts about Adam's apple, lasting for several weeks, which is capable of producing consumption or death in any manner.

The voice is affected in every degree, from a slight hoarseness to complete loss of voice, with a feeling sometimes, of rasping, rawness, or burning.

Some compare the pain to the sensation of a sore; others to a pricking, or a heat in the throat, or side of the neck, sometimes both sides of the neck at the bottom, about half way between the shoulder and top of the breast bone.

In advanced stages there is difficulty of swallowing, and drinks return by the nose.

Dr. Stokes says: "In some it is traceable to a syphilitic origin; in others to a scrofulous; in a third from inflammation in an apparently uncontaminated constitution.

A sticky, tough substance, sometimes gathers on the back part of the throat, occasioning the most distressing fits of coughing, which is often decided to be beginning consumption; when a week or two of proper treatment restores to usual health.

When the disease is beginning, there is no feeling of pain or soreness, but a frequent disposition to hem, or hawk, or clear the throat, especially just before beginning to speak. When any thing is brought away by these efforts, it is at first a clear, pearly looking, gluey feeling substance, which, as the disease progresses, becomes yellow, dark or greenish, especially in the morning; constantly, though very slowly getting worse, in the progress of weeks, months or years; now and then terminating in sudden death. In my experience, none of these cases, especially if accompanied by a pricking sensation in the throat, or swallowing, or turning the head, ever get well of themselves.

For the still more perfect understanding of my meaning on several points, I here propose a few inquiries, and append my answers:

When is a man threatened with Consumption?

Ans. If a man ever spits up red blood, even to the amount of half a teaspoonful, coming up with a slight tickle in the throat or short heck of a cough, he will in nine cases out of ten, die of Consumption, sooner or later, however perfect he may appear in health in every respect,

Ans. 2. If a man has a slight heck or cough every morning on getting up, for weeks together, or on lying down at night, or both, he will, in nine cases out of ten, die of consumption, sooner or later, however perfect he may be in health in every other respect. In either case acute disease excepted.

When has a man actual Consumption of the Lungs?

Ans. A man has actual Consumption when he has a cough night and morning; pulse always above ninety; a heavy yellow expectoration; cold sweats towards morning, bowels too loose or too costive; frequently restless, unrefreshing sleep; variable appetite; weakness about the legs and knees; shortness of breath in going up stairs, or walking up hill; falling away; general feeling of weakness and lassitude; but little disposition to move about; soft and flabby muscles in the arms and legs. A man who has these symptoms has Consumption, and it is impossible for it to be anything else but Consumption; and his lungs are rotting away every hour. More! He has Consumption, if he has the majority of those symptoms.

What do you mean by the cure of Consumption?

Ans. If a man comes to me with a bad cough, pains about the breast, irregular bowels, variable appetite, short breath, night sweats, rapid pulse, "falling off," and goes away without any of these things, and at the end of one, two, or three years, I meet him on the street, or he comes to see me, and says he has no cough, no pain, sleeps sound, bowels regular, never takes any medicine, and weighs as much as ever he did in his life; I say such a man is cured of Consumption. Such were No. One, page thirty-seven: No. Six, page forty-seven; Nos. 2, 3, 4, and 5, page forty-nine; case A, page 148; case B, page 149; case A, page 174; and others not necessary to be named. I hope to be able to accomplish the same again.

When is a man threatened with fatal disease, called by the various names of Bronchitis, Clergyman's Sore Throat, and Throat Consumption?

Ans. He is thus threatened if he has any alteration of voice for several weeks, with a frequent disposition to clear the throat, and slight soreness or swelling, or pricking, in pressing the front or sides of Adam's apple, or in swallowing.

When has a man this so called Bronchitis, and this only, and cannot have Consumption at the same time?

Ans. If he have chronic hoarseness, pain or soreness on pressing the throat, with a frequent feeling of dryness, general health good, bowels, appetite, sleep, pretty regular, with a pulse under 72 at all times—this is Bronchitis, so called, and it is impossible for it at this stage, to be complicated with Consumption.

When is such a man cured?

Ans. He is cured when he has no pricking, dryness, smarting, or heating sensation about the throat at any time; has no hoarseness of the voice, and can speak as loud and long as others without unusual effort of fatigue.

Having been successful in accomplishing these objects in a variety of cases, I shall rest with having stated the fact, leaving it with those who are unfortunately affected in this manner, to adopt the means proposed, or seek for others.

I am extremely gratified in being able to state, that the cases of Consumption which I published several years ago as cured by me, are yet, as far as I know, alive and well, thus establishing the truth of the permanency of the cures performed.

No. One, 2, page 37, called at my office last week. I had not seen him for near four years. He was well, looked well, and felt well in every respect; was on his way to New Orleans in July, and had no apprehensions of sickness. As far as his appearance to others, and his feelings to himself, there was not the vestige of any disease, any where about him.

This gentleman also informed me that case Three, 16, page 47, was the healthy, happy mother of two fine children.

Case Four, page 46, Perfectly well. Case Six, 37—and others I could name, but it is not necessary.

Case Eight, page 48, is not only well, but has cleared in legitimate business, since I cured him, twenty-eight thousand dollars; and thinks nothing, at the age of fifty-three, of galloping forty miles, from New Orleans to his sugar plantation, *after sundown.*

The lawyer, on page 121, is now, at the end of three years, a hale, hearty, healthy man, as I learned two days ago, from a neighbor of his, who has come a thousand miles for the removal of a throat affection, and I greatly hope his journey will be re-measured in health and happiness.

I doubt not many of those cases which have been named are doing well; but living in different and distant parts of the country, my opportunities of hearing from them are occasional and accidental. The case, for example, on page 49, has, after the interval of another year, reported himself "as well as he ever was."

The great, the main object in preparing these pages, is, as has been repeatedly named, to enable persons to understand what are the feelings and symptoms which generally bring on and accompany consumption; and to induce them to apply, without delay, for their prompt and effectual removal; believing as I do, in the uniform certainty of its accomplishment, under the conditions named, and that it would be the means every year of saving from a premature and fearful death, many thousands of the kindliest and loveliest of our race.

ILLUSTRATION.

A young lady, aged eighteen, of uncommon personal beauty, attended by her mother, desired an examination, in great apprehension, that the lungs were affected. During the preceding twelve months she had been prescribed for, at different times, by a very distinguished surgeon. She complained of constant headache; cold feet; heavy pain at the pit of the stomach; great chilliness; "a pestersome dry cough at times;" pains through the breast and sides; sometimes a feeling of soreness in the right side; indisposed to exercise; variable appetite; had spitting of blood on several occasions. Within three weeks every symptom was removed, and, as far as I know, she remains well to this day. There can be no doubt that had these complaints been unheeded, she would finally have fallen into a fatal decline; and yet it is seen with what comparative ease she has recovered from symptoms well calculated to alarm.

TO MOTHERS.

Many young girls, just rising into womanhood, become listless and inattentive; lose their liveliness; sit about the house, taking little interest in what is going on around them; do not appear to eat anything; lie in bed late in the morning; and when they do come down, seem more dead than alive, occasional pains about the breast and shoulders; complain of much chilliness, if the weather is but a little cold. Such persons are unfeelingly accused of *laziness; of having the blues;* that they *don't need any thing;* and not being sympathized with, they keep their ailments to themselves, and suffer pain in silence rather than run the risk of an unfeeling contradiction; and many times, when it is too late, it is decided that *something must be done.* In a majority of these cases, the cough is not noticed by others, for it is but slight; occurring only on lying down, or getting up, and lasts but a minute or two. In all these cases an unnatural pulse, short or quick breathing, with a deficient action of the lungs are always present, to a greater or less extent. By a neglect of these considerations, parents have suffered many a bitter pang, and spent many an hour in unavailing chiding and self-reproach, when the object, around which their memories gather can receive their cares no more. A beautiful flower never droops without an adequate cause; and whenever a youthful heart is listless and sad, there is always occasion for it, and whether imaginary or real, it ought to be removed by kindness, sympathy, and skill.

In some cases, Consumption, Bronchitis, and Laryngitis, have so many symptoms in common, as to mislead and baffle the skill of the most eminent physicians. But these ailments have become so frequent and uniformly fatal, that the necessity of studying and endeavoring to discriminate them, has forced itself on the minds of medical men, and the results have been gratifying in the extreme. The difference between these diseases has been made so apparent; the modes of treatment are so diverse and novel; while the practical results have become so manifest and important, in restoring eminent public men to usefulness, who had abandoned their professional occupations in despair, that it is a pleasure to invoke publicity, and call the attention of all, to the study of the subject, the new modes of treatment, and their successful issue.

These pages are prepared, not to instruct the common reader how he may cure himself, but to enable him to discriminate these dangerous diseases, and know for himself whether he has Bronchitis, Consumption, or Laryngitis; and having determined this most essential point, to apply, without delay, for appropriate treatment. The three ailments just mentioned are so mixed up in the minds of men, there is such a limited understanding of what they really are, that persons sometimes come to me, after studying and enquiring, perhaps for months together, with the wish to comprehend the nature of their sickness; and in a manner and tone indicating perfect hopelessness of ever being able to understand the subject, ask with great eagerness and earnestness: *"Doctor, what is the matter with me? some say I have incipient consumption; others, that it is only an attack of Bronchitis. What is Bronchitis? Are my lungs affected or not?"* In such a frame of mind, many persons apply to a physician; but even if he give a favorable opinion, they feel themselves perfectly in the dark; and the tormenting thought is still suggested: *"He knows it is Consumption, but does not like to tell me?"* Then he begins to reconsider his symptoms; he is thrown anew into a state of feverish disquietude, and cannot rest until he asks the advice of another physician. The reader of these pages, who has some suspicion that his own lungs are affected, will feel more deeply than any language of mine can express, the full import of the oft repeated apostrophe, in burning thoughts, if not in audible speech: *"I would give anything in the world to know really whether I have the Consumption or not!"* The agonizing desire to have this question truthfully and satisfactorily settled, arises from the general belief that it is a question of life and death: for the thought has almost become instinctive: *"If it is Consumption, I may as well make up my mind to die."* Under circumstances of so much doubt and perplexity, and, at the same time, so momentous, I cannot but think that the new means which I propose of deciding in any one case: "It is not Consumption, it is impossible;" or, "It is Consumption, so far advanced, that in your case, recovery is hopeless, and your death within a very few weeks is inevitable;"—must be looked upon with the deepest interest; especially, as they afford strictly demonstrative proof as to the three points following:—

If all of a man's lungs are within him,—if he has lost none of them by decay,— if there be no consuming process going on there, this important fact is indicated with great certainty, in spite of every symptom, feeling, and appearance to the contrary; by which I mean to say, that if a man can come up to the physical requisitions of this new mode of diagnosis, it is utterly impossible that the lungs should be in a state of decay; that any of them should have been lost.

A second fact, arrived at with mathematical precision, is, that when a man's lungs are in a state of decay, when there is even a small cavity, it is physically impossible for him to come up to the physical requisitions.

The third point of interest is, thet the proportion of a man's lungs lost by decay, or rendered otherwise inoperative, is indicated to a fraction of the one two-hundredth part of the whole.

In this new mode of determining the condition of the lungs, nothing is left to the mere opinion of the physician, or the hopes or wishes of the patient. If all a man's lungs are within him, if there is no decay, he can know it for himself, and no man can mislead him. Auscultation, and percussion, and plessimetry may deceive, and have deceived medical men of the highest eminence; but in these new means, in conjunction with auscultation, there can be no mistake, there can be no deception as to either of the three points above named.

This new method of diagnosis is invaluable as to two other points: it indicates a man's improvement, irrespective of symptoms, feelings and appearances; but when the patient is dying by piece-meal, however well he may feel, and however often he may say, "I'm better," no dial plate ever indicated more certainly the passing hour, than these means do, that his life is rapidly passing away.

There is, furthermore, a practical advantage derived from this new diagnostic, which is beyond all price; it does what is claimed for no other method, to-wit: discovers the existence of consumption in its earliest forming stages, long before the slightest decay has taken place; and. by thus indicating its early presence, before it has fixed itself in the system, a timely warning is given, and consumption becomes one of the most manageable diseases; for, however incurable it is generally considered, in its advanced stages, that is, when the lungs have already begun to decay and rot away, there is perhaps no one so ill informed, as to deny that it may be warded off, if attempted at an early stage, before decay has set in.

It is my opinion, that four persons out of five could be saved from falling victims to consumptive disease, were my plan of treatment begun and carried out, perseveringly and energetically, as soon of the means proposed, in conjunction with auscultation, indicate the commencement of consumption. Auscultation corroborates, as far as it goes, but these new means indicate the existence of phthisis at a stage far, very far in advance of stethescopy.

Much more might be said in praise of this new method of investigation, but I choose to leave the more demonstrative developments to time, lest what I say be deemed so extravagant as to frighten away inquiry. It is my belief that a happier thought never occurred in medicine, saving the praises due to Hervey and Jenner. It is my purpose to make a full publication hereafter, when a greater variety of facts, bearing on the subject, have been collected, and when more leisure is afforded for reducing it to a system, by which it may be rendered safe and practically and generally useful. In this simple tract, for general distribution, I did not design anything beyond a bare allusion to the subject, and a few illustrations of its practical utility.

Persons have often come to me, believing themselves, believed by their friends, and pronounced by physicians, to have actual consumption; yet the means referred to, have enabled me promptly to say, "you have no consumption—it cannot be;" and their rapid and permanent recovery, by the use of authorized means, as indicated by what are allowed to be the general principles of medicine, has fully confirmed the truth of my opinion; and it is to the partiality of these persons, and their friends, that I am indebted to a reported ability in the treatment of consumption, not altogether due to me.

WHAT I BELIEVE.

I believe in the cure of consumption, prompt, perfect and permanent, if attempted before it is fixed in the system; and believing this, I have, for a series of years, applied myself to the employment of means to find out. more certainly, what were the signs and symptoms given in the more early stages of the terrible malady. Medical men, and others, universally admit that consumption might be cured if proper efforts were made at the early onset of the disease; but it is as universally acknowledged, that there are no certain means of ascertaining its presence in the forming stages; and this is equivalent to admitting that "Consumption cannot be cured, and it is not worth while to try;" a theory which has been practically carried out by old and young to the present time. I believe that consumption, like cholera, is fatal in its last stages, but entirely manageable if attempted the moment the premonitory symptoms manifest themselves. I have endeavored to find out what the premonitory symptoms of Consumption are, and by the aid of men and books and instruments, I think I have attained the knowledge at once so desirable and so vitally important; a knowledge which, I fully believe, will rescue many from an untimely grave.

I have observed what no physician of ordinary capacity could help from observing, that in the last stages of Consumption, the heart and lungs work too fast by one half. This increased action comes on by the slowest, almost imperceptible degrees; never suddenly in a day, or week or month; but there is a time when the first departure is made from the natural standard; and there are other symptoms which as invariably attend this state of things, as a shadow attends a body in sun-light; and more—these symptoms, when connected with this increased activity, never fail to end in death by consumption, in its most unmistakable form, if appropriate efforts are not promptly and perseveringly made to remove them at this early stage of their development. The most prominent of these symptoms are—loss of strength, loss of breath on exercising, and loss of flesh; the bowels as yet being regular, sleep sound, appetite good: the almost only symptom appreciable to the patient being a cough, or heck, or hem, so slight and seldom at first, as to attract no notice. But when it comes to a hacking or cough every night on lying down, or every morning on getting up, it should excite the liveliest alarm. By following up the inquiries and making a free use of the knowledge and investigations and experience of others, however obscure and humble their position in society, for truth is truth, whether from a gutter or a university, I think I have arrived at results of the most important character in their bearings on the health and happiness and lives of my fellow race.

Physiologists say that a man's height equals his measurement from tip to tip of the fingers, when the arms are extended. It is also affirmed, that the length of a man's intestines, are five times the length of his body.

Why may not the amount of a man's lungs, when in free and healthful operation, bear a definite and unvarying relation to some of his physical proportions? It will occur at once to the reader, that the amount of a man's lungs depends on the size of his breast, measuring around the body; but such is not the fact. Under certain limitations, not as yet fully defined, it is found that the amount of a healthy man's lungs depends on fixed physical conditions—the height, weight, age, sex, degree of health, arterial and respiratory action. The height is the predominant guide, other things being equal. Beginning at five feet, the increase of lung measurement is eight times the increase in height. With this data, it is easy to ascertain the healthy measurement of every individual. And by making several thousand experiments, taking the measurement and other physical conditions into account in each case, this important point is arrived at with admirable and arithmetical certainly, how much should a man's lungs measure in perfect health in every respect, of certain physical conditions. If in a thousand successive cases, I find that every healthy man of the requisite physical conditions, gives precisely the same measurement, I conclude that any one who does not come up to that measurement, has just that amount of deficiency of lung action. If a man in perfect health of lungs measures two hundred, it is easy to see, that if half his lungs are gone, he will measure only half as much: and so with any other larger or smaller proportion, *down to one cubic inch!*

PRACTICAL RESULTS.

The actual practical results correspond with the above statements. A man came into my office who had lost half his measurement. I told his brother that although appearances were against the opinion I was going to give, and he had walked to my office from his own apartments, several squares off, without much fatigue, yet I felt bound to say he could not survive three weeks. Within that time he died with unmistakable consumption.

Another gentleman came to me from North Alabama attended by his brother, who was extremely anxious to know his condition, but desired me to withhold my opinion from the invalid. He told me his brother had been improving of late, and was greatly better and stronger and livelier than he had been for some time past. On examination, I found he had lost two-fifths of his measurement; and I felt compelled to say, that he could not under any conceivable circumstances live six weeks, and that he ought to be taken to his family without the least delay. He died in about five weeks from that time. These are given as examples from many others. In short, the use which I make of these things is simply this,—if a man is deficient in measurement,and under my treatment, he lessens that deficiency every week, I encourage him to persevere, for he is evidently and substantially improving. If, unfortunately, on the other hand, the deficiency increases every week, notwithstanding all I can do, I send him home, because he is declining every day, and must inevitably die; and I desire to receive money from no man unless I believe that I am doing him a commensurate good. A physician of extensive practice and good family, from Kentucky, called to see me. I explained every thing to him as fully as I could, and on submitting himself to examination, he said at once, in a manner and tone so despairing and melancholy, that I can never forget, "*I see it—it is no use to try any thing; I may as well go home and die.*" He started on his return the next morning, and died not long after his arrival. With facts like these, constantly occurring, I look upon this new diagnostic with increasing admiration.

A deficiency of measurement arises from two principal causes.

An actual loss of the substance of the lungs; or an infiltration, or engorgement or solidification. Auscultation must decide which of these it is. A young gentleman came to me from one of the western counties of Missouri. He was sent by an elder brother who had been cured by me, of cough, pain in the breast, &c., several years before. His principal symptoms were distressing pains about the breast, no appetite, sleepless nights, and such an inveterate spitting of blood, that walking two or three squares would cause him to bring it up by mouthfuls. His deficiency of lung measurement was nearly one third: but auscultation showed that it came from the air cells of the lungs being filled up with collections that did not properly belong there. His brother was greatly alarmed: his family physician said it was no use for him to come to me, as it was a clear case of tubercular consumption. I at once informed his brother that I thought he could be cured, and that so far from its being a dangerous case, that he could safely and profitably leave for home in a week. I gave him some vegetable pills, administered quinine and elixir of vitriol three times a day, and required him to walk about the city from morning till night; never carrying his exercise to fatigue or exhaustion. Within a week he ceased to spit blood altogether; his appetite returned, his sleep became sound, unbroken and refreshing; his bowels regular daily, without medicine for that purpose; whereas, before, they had kept obstinately costive; his strength returned so that he could walk for hours at a time without special fatigue; and on the eight day when he left, his lungs measured to the full healthy standard. With results like these, I should be excused if I speak enthusiastically in these pages. These are facts, and I consider them triumphant. And in recording them I enjoy that pleasurable feeling which a man possesses, when he knows he is right, and yet sees that the multitude now incredulous, will sooner or later agree with him.

In confirmation of my views in relation to the importance and value of this new method of determining the actual condition of the lungs, what proportion of them are in healthful and efficient operation, I will give the testimony of two of the most respectable and extensive periodicals in the world. The London Lancet, one of whose Editors has been for some years a member of the British Parliament, and who is honored every session by appointments on committees, among the most important to a nation's interests, says: "This mode of distinguishing Consumption at an earlier period than by any other means, has been actually proved."

The British and Foreign Medical Review, now edited by Dr. Forbes; and which has been conducted with such signal ability for the last quarter of a century, that it is now circulated in every quarter of the globe, says: "We have no hesitation in recording our deliberate opinion that this is one of the most valuable contributions to physiological science that we have met with for some time." I consider the stethescope and percussion as mere toys, which do well enough to excite the wonder of the credulous. I must confess they never gave me any satisfaction. I never could learn anything by them. It may be different with others, but I believe that the ear laid upon the patient's breast, with nothing intervening but a single thickness of the inner garment, stretched without a wrinkle and laid smoothly on the skin, is immeasurably preferable to any stethescope ever invented, it tells us more certainly and in louder tones by far, all that stethescopy and percussion pretend to, and in a more simple and natural manner. In all cases I use the ear directly, to ascertain the more prominent sounds, but the stethescope and percussion never, except for a single reason, and that does not occur once in a hundred cases; nor do I place any dependence on the eye, nor the moving of the extended hand over the chest. In forming an opinion in a case of Consumption, the main foundations are,

The condition of the pulse.

The degree of the emaciation.

The measurement of, the lungs.

The sounds given to the ear when it is laid on the patient's breast, while standing; or back while stooping forward; a single thickness only intervening of the inner garment stretched smoothly over the skin. The cough, spitting of blood, and that which is expectorated, I consider, of themselves, of little consequence, for the simple reason that they never can be relied upon, until a stage so late, that no reliance is needed. No one pretends that either of them have an invariable cause, an invariable effect, or an invariable tendency, therefore, by themselves, they are symptoms of little value.

UNSEEN CASES.

Some of the most gratifying, and remarkable cures I have ever performed, in cases of Throat disease and Consumption, have been of persons whom I have never seen, or have seen but once: this arises from the fact, that any one of observation, by confining himself to a certain class of diseases for a series of years, acquires an ability almost instinctive, to determine the value of symptoms arising in a certain order; and in their progress, attended by certain changes; and the blank form which I send to those at a distance, who cannot conveniently come to me, enable me to trace the order, and the progress and the changes of these symptoms with great facility. And then, there are two inestimable advantages in being prescribed for in such cases.—The patient is at home, the very last place for an invalid to leave, except for a very few days at a time, a truth seldom learned except by experience gained in bitterness and unavailing tears.

By being away from his physician, a thousand minor ailments are left to take care of themselves, and do so better than by a physician's aid, while the main course of treatment goes on steadily, uninterruptedly, and in a determined and business like manner without the worse than leaden draw backs, of being in a large city, on expenses, among strangers, nothing tó do, no where to go, and nobody to talk to. An invalid from the country soon finds that a city is the most lonely place in the world to be at; no body has time to talk to him, for talk's sake. The city in summer is an oven; and if you walk or ride for fresh air, you must go through miles of dust, and what is worse—*return* through the same. In winter you are in an everlasting fog of coal dust, and there is no way of getting rid of it but through miles of mud.

When persons have disease of the Throat, and not Consumption, they express themselves in different ways, in describing their ailment, such as tired, pricking, heavy aching, scraping, dry, raw, choking, tickling. Some refer these feelings to the region of Adam's apple; and others to the little hollow at the bottom of the neck, just above the breast bone. Some complain of a burning sensation at the top of the breast bone, others at the centre. A great many complain of some disagreeable feeling at the pit of the stomach. One man says he is all the time hawking, and brings up little or nothing: another is constantly swallowing, but as soon as the swallowing is over, the feeling returns; this is very much the sensation some persons have, after swallowing a pill, feeling as if it were but half way down. Sometimes this sensation arises from the palate being relaxed; at others, from great inflammation at the back part of the throat, by which a clear glairy, sticky, or yellowish matter is thrown off, but as soon as it is hawked away or swallowed, more collects, and thus the person is constantly carrying this disagreeable stuff into the stomach, among the food, and in time his appetite becomes impaired, the coats of the stomach injured, and a species of dispepsia originated, with all its train of disagreeable, disheartening symptoms of bad taste in the mouth, irregular appetite, a tiredness of feeling all over the body, no disposition to do anything, low spirits; and in time the person becomes silent, moody, and melancholy, and loses all his energy and ambition. In such cases nothing can be done, until the dyspepsia is removed, which is often accomplished in a short time, and then the throat is cured without any trouble by a few daily applications of the argentine solution, and the use of the simple gargles.

Many persons have come to me who had had the uvula cut off, but scarcely ever have I seen a person who could say, decidedly, that it had been of any material advantage. Some think that they were a little better for a while, but the great majority "didn't see that it did them any good." In all the cases that have applied to me, I have never yet had occasion to take off the palate, but always succeeded in causing it to contract, by the use of the simple gargles. And since the cutting off of a palate has sometimes been the occasion of a great deal of suffering, especially if enough has not been taken off, I prefer avoiding the risk, and by curing it with gargles, leaving it in its natural state, I have never yet failed. Still it may be sometimes necessary.

APPARENT CONSUMPTION.

There can be no doubt that many persons are wrongfully pronounced to be in Consumption, from a want of proper knowledge and skill, on the part of the person giving the opinion, thereby throwing the patient into hopeless melancholy, or abandoning him to palliative means, and neglecting a course of treatment, which, with more truthful views, would have saved him.

A CASE.

A Southern planter, of great wealth and distinction, called upon me, on his way to the West Indies, in pursuit of health. His prevailing symptoms were a most incessant cough, day and night; it had taken away his appetite and sleep; he had been a large portly man, but had fallen off so much that his skin was wrinkled, and his clothing appeared lost on him; he was haggard and dispirited in the extreme. He had night sweats, and a constant, fixed pain in the centre of the breast. His friends had given him up. His banker said to me, in a very cold, business-like, confident way—"He is too far gone to be saved. Do you think you will be able to do the old gentleman any good?" His family scarcely expect to see him return. He was very costive, and complained much of debility; that his coughing and expectoration weakened him very much. His tongue was dry and furred, and he was very much troubled with shortness of breath   Conversation, exercise, going up stairs, coming into a room from out doors, invariably excited a most distressing dry cough, and he had no appetite for anything. His pulse was ninety-five a minute. Upon examination, I gave my unhesitating opinion, that his was not a case of consumption. This opinion gave him great uneasiness, for he had evidently come to me with high expectations, and that I should give such an opinion, in the face of what every body believed, himself included, caused him to apprehend that I did not understand his disease, and of course could do him no good; it was like abandoning a last hope of life. Had I told him at once, that it was a plain case of Consumption, but that I would certainly cure him in a short time, he would have been much better satisfied. He had a great many questions, unanswerable, as he imagined, to propose to me. How is it that I cough so much? Where do these night sweats come from? If my lungs are not diseased, how is it that I have this incessant pain in the breast? If my lungs are not giving way, why have I fallen off so much, and have such shortness of breath, that I am tired to death when I go up stairs? Every day or two he wanted me to examine him again, saying he was afraid I had made a mistake. To all this I replied, that his was a clear case of Throat disease, and that he would soon be satisfied of that fact. I made daily applications to his throat, for several weeks, and by properly regulating the general system, I find an entry in my note book, some eight weeks afterwards to this effect:

"Returned in good health and fine spirits; appetite excellent; sleep is delicious, without any artificial means; breathing sixteen; pulse seventy-two; natural ruddiness returned to him; sleeps on either side with perfect ease, which has not been done for a long time before; not the slightest remnant of pain in the breast, for the last month; weariness in walking, and shortness of breath have entirely disappeared.

In this case, the cough was not entirely removed, which was attributable to a singular accident which had befallen him, and which would probably cause some cough, as long as he lived; but not sufficient to make it necessary to take anything for it, or to be called troublesome. At the same time, I believe, if he could have been induced to live on plain diet, and to leave off the use of tobacco altogether, the remnant of cough would soon entirely disappear. The immoderate use of tobacco, by smoking or chewing, is a cause of disease of the throat, in a number of instances; and whether a cause or not, a perfect cure is almost impossible, unless it is wholly abandoned, in every shape and form.

For the benefit of such as may not be able to obtain the larger publication, I will state a few cases, showing how many of the symptoms of consumption, persons may have, and yet the lungs be entirely sound; and showing, at the same time, the necessity of applying to competent and experienced persons to decide so important a question.

A female, aged thirty, was very subject to taking cold; this ended in spitting blood, and great difficulty in breathing; pain in the throat; a hoarse voice; frequent pulse; and night sweats; she died in six months, and on opening the body the lungs were found to be entirely healthy, and the whole disease seated in the larynx and windpipe.

A man, aged thirty, very liable to take cold, had been sick a long time; considerable spitting of blood, at different times; face lean; loss of voice; painful and fatiguing cough; brings up mucus and yellow matter; obstinate diarrhœa. He died; the three last days being passed in extreme suffering and agony. On opening the breast, the lungs presented no unusual appearance. The disease was at the upper part of the windpipe, which was ulcerated.

A youth, of eighteen, had pain in the throat; voice changed; spit up sometimes mouthfuls of frothy red blood; frequent general chills; great falling off; pale and sharp features; cheeks red; spit up lumps of yellow matter; frequent pulse; night sweats; difficult breathing; and death within a year. On opening his body, there was found no ulceration in the lungs, but the upper part of the windpipe, about the voice-making organs, was ulcerated.

A man, aged forty-nine, had a harsh dry cough; expectorated a whitish, thick stuff, sometimes with blood, frothy, with little masses of matter scattered through it. He died, but no tubercles were found in the lungs.

A boy, of fifteen became addicted to bad habits, in four years he began to experience pain in the throat; the voice altered, became shrill at first, and was then entirely lost; swallowing liquids became impossible; he expectorated large quantities of matter, and died after a year's illness. The lungs were found entirely sound, but the whole throat was ulcerated.

In stubborn cases of throat disease, it is sometimes necessary to prohibit for awhile the marital rights. Cases are given in books where throat ail has followed excessive indulgencies within a few hours, and ultimate death, with ordinary symptoms of of consumption, without the lungs being implicated in any way. These facts demand the consideration of all.

There is a disease, called by different names, to-wit;—Throat-ail, Bronchitis, Clergyman's Sore Throat, where there is frequent swallowing, clearing the throat, pricking sensation, more or less hoarseness or loss of voice, so as not to be able to speak above a whisper, or spells of difficult breathing. This disease has one or more of these symptoms. It is very fatal, often suddenly so, at midnight, from suffocation. This ailment is easily cured. Sometimes the voice is restored within a week, after having been lost for months; at other times, several months are required. Little or no internal medicine is used, and there is no confinement to the house or detention from business. This Throat-ail sometimes gives all the more prominent symptoms of Consumption, such as an incessant hacking cough, pain in the breast, sleepless nights, great falling away, weakness, spitting blood, and night sweats; and yet the lungs be perfectly sound, for the patient has recovered rapidly and completely, without the use of a particle of the ordinary medicine used in Consumption. I wish a knowledge of this fact could be spread from Maine to Florida; and from New England to Oregon.

A CASE.

Last year a gentleman of fortune, aged fifty-one, was talking in a stage coach, and felt a sudden giving away of something in his throat. He became alarmed, and applied to his old neighbor and friend, a professor in the medical school, who assured him he would be well in three days. A dozen leeches were applied to his throat, and several blisters; and being no better at the end of three weeks he applied to me. I could only hear him speak by placing my ear to his lips. Within a week, he could speak in his natural tone of voice, without effort or injury; and left my office CURED, *and remains so to this day.*

A clergyman had given up preaching for many months; after the fourth application he said, "I enjoy the luxury of a full breath, which I have not done for many a long day before." In two weeks he preached without any special inconvenience, and as far as I know, has had no return of his malady.

One of the loveliest and most beautiful young women of this city lost her voice—she had not spoken above a whisper for three months; at the fourth application she spoke in a loud tone, overwhelmed with gladness.

A case is reported of a young lady from South Carolina, who had not spoken above a whisper for nine months, and supposed her voice irrecoverably gone; at the fifth application she arose from her seat, bathed in tears of gratitude, *speaking in her natural tone!!*—It must not be forgotten, however, that some cases require applications extended through months.

These applications afford instant relief in the croup of young children. There is another species of Throat-ail in children.

Mrs. M.'s little daughter, aged seven years, seldom laid down in her bed—the mother was in constant fear of suffocation; this extended throughout months. She called to me in great distress—the difficulty was removed in ten minutes, and never returned.—Miss M. E. S., a beautiful little girl, often woke her parents in the night, by the noise of her suffocative breathing. She was brought to my office, and was relieved *beyond recurrence,* in three minutes.

When ulceration has attacked the organs of voice and eaten them away; or when the vocal chords have shrunken or dried up, there is no cure; nor when there is necrosis or a destruction of the bones or cartilages of the part.

When the ulceration has been neglected, and has extended below the forks of the windpipe, which is just behind the top of the breast bone, the patient must die in a short time, because the applications cannot be made below the hollow at the bottom of the neck in front, and the parts are soon eaten through: a speedy death is inevitable.

By reference to page *twenty-two,* the reader will perceive how uniformly these slight throat affections, and from trivial causes, go on to a painful and fatal termination. A few other cases are here given from a foreign publication:

A physician was called to ride on a January night, and contracted a hoarseness, which continued with very little cough and no expectoration; his general health continued excellent; no one could have supposed anything the matter with him. His voice became more and more hoarse, until it was entirely lost, and in a few months afterwards he died.

A lady was attacked with fits of dry cough, and subsequently lost her voice; there was a sense of scraping in the throat; sometimes obstinate sneezing; the cough was a little soothed by drinking water; the breathing gradually became difficult, swallowing painful, and she died.

A gentleman observed for a year past, that his voice was occasionally a little cracked, and soon became permanently hoarse, and at last it was entirely lost. There was no pain, no swelling, no spitting of blood; he seemed to enjoy the fullest health; yet the symptoms gradually grew worse until he died.

I trust that the record of these cases will be a warning to those who have any ailment in the throat, and that they will be induced to take prompt measures for the effectual eradication of the disease.

The statements made in these pages are founded on my own personal observation, and being convinced of their truth myself, I simply record the facts, and trust to their reasonableness for convincing the common-sense reader.

FALSE IMPRESSIONS.

I do not wish to leave an impression on the mind of any one, that I am every year curing thousands who were in the last stages of consumption ; all such statements carry with them their own absurdity and recklessness : if the reader is unfortunately in the last stages of Consumption, I would make no effort to convince him that I could cure him, but would sooner counsel him to prepare at once, if he has been so unwise as to neglect it hitherto, for the great untried future, upon which the most healthy of us must so soon enter. I would rather inform him that recovery from the last stages of the Consumption does sometimes occur, and the person dies many years afterwards of some totally different disease—but that this happens so rarely it should be considered an exception rather than a rule, a thing never to be promised, and seldom to he hoped for.

WHAT I DO.

I, however, do labor to show how certainly I can detect Consumption in its first forming stages, and with what comparative ease, and how promptly and effectually it can be warded off, and the constitution placed in a healthy condition, in many instances. I feel quite sure this could be done in four cases out of five; and the success which has been attributed to me in the treatment of Consumption, is due to my being able to detect it, in its first forming stages, in its very first approaches ; and not only to detect it, but to prove its early presence most satisfactorily ; not, indeed, by mere reasoning and theory, but by bringing to light physical signs and symptoms, which rationality cannot resist.

Any success which I may have had, is not the result of wonder-working medical compounds, for I administer but little medicine for the consumption itself ; nor have any cures performed by me, been the result of ingeniously contrived patented instruments. Long experience, and extended observation, have convinced me, and are daily confirming me in the conviction that patented contrivances for the alleviation of human suffering, are too often founded in heartless cupidity ; for who, that possesses any generosity, would say to a suffering, perishing fellow creature : *this contrivance of mine will restore you to health, but if you make one yourself, I will imprison or ruin you by a law suit, and unless you buy one of mine, you may suffer on, and perish.* Such, it appears to me, is the language of every man who patents a remedy for the removal of human suffering, and the same of those who deal in them.

FEMALES.

Women are liable to throat diseases, from three causes :
Suppression of monthly turns.
Damp or cold feet.
Dyspepsia or Indigestion.
In this last case the stomach, liver and bowels must be brought into a healthy condition, with the use of as little medicine as possible, and daily applications must be made to the parts, until they are restored.

When suppression is the cause, a restoration of a clear voice is not to be expected until regularity is established.

In either case if neglected, the malady makes a steady and often hidden progress, and, sooner or later, ends in a fatal form of disease.

MY OPINION.

I am often asked : Do you approve of supporters or braces? I believe that such contrivances are unnatural, irrational, mischievous and absurd. No one part of the body can be supported by pressure, unless by imposing a greater strain on some other part than was designed by nature, and that other part must suffer sooner or later, if the extra burden is continued. Nature is free in all her operations, and any contrivances which impede the natural freedom of bodily motion, must be mischievous, if persevered in. Numbers have come to me, after having obtained these things at considerable expense and trouble, uniformly giving testimony to their utter inefficiency when worn; or their inability to wear them without producing greater ills than those originally complained of. In some instances they may be of service. I have known no such instance as yet. I will state a simple fact, officially reported, and leave the reader, to judge for himself, and not to submit to the persuasions of those whose interest it is to sell these things, and who may sincerely believe all they say; but the question arises, "Is it true?" Your money, your health, your life, are the issues, and you are most interested in forming a correct judgment.

A large portion of British soldiers, who enlisted at the age of eighteen years, were noticed to die within five years of Consumption. Such an appalling fact elicited the closest scrutiny, and it was attributed to the weight of the knapsack pressing on the shoulders, on the whole upper part of the breast, where the decay of common Consumption always begins; and continued pressure at any point about the shoulders or breast, will excite or hasten the disease. This is a bare fact, which no assertion can explain away. And the reader should bear in mind always, that the only natural, healthful condition of the body, is a condition of unrestraint. Nature no more "abhors a vacuum," than confinement, even for a moment. I have never yet known a person to obtain a bandage or supporter, or braces for the lungs, that did not soon throw them away; sometimes within twenty-four hours of their purchase; and repeatedly within two weeks.

Patent medicines are liable to the same, and even greater objections; for while it is asserted by traffickers in them, that they are so simple that they cannot possibly do any harm, even if they do no good, it is known to every observant physician, that in many instances they have a most pernicious effect; oftentimes destroying the tone of the stomach for life, and poisoning the whole system. An article taken by the "HOME JOURNAL," from a London paper, contains a just satire, headed:

MORTALITY FOR THE MILLION.

The Earl of Harrowby is reported to have stated at a meeting of the society for the Promotion of Colonization, that "the population is increasing at the rate of one thousand souls a day. It cannot be said that the government is doing nothing to supply a remedy for this monster evil; for government sanctions the sale of quack medicines, than which nothing can operate more effectually as a check to over-pop-ulation."

It cannot be denied that drugs, and drops, and syrups, and balms and balsams are too freely resorted to, and too lavishly used among all classes of society, even among the better informed, and I here give as an example of their pernicious ten-dency, the following item going the newspaper rounds:—

"The editor of the Boston Chronotype, who lost several children by administering to them patent medicines for summer diseases, has since treated the same complaints successfully, by giving ice and iced water, and recommends this substitute to others. The relief it grants is gradual and certain."

Here is a case of an intelligent man, in a responsible official station, in the most learned city in the nation, becoming, to a certain extent, the destroyer of his children, by giving them medicines about which he knew nothing, except the assertion of those whose interest it was to sell them. How many lives might be preserved, and how many good constitutions saved from wreck and ruin, if the people generally would learn a lesson from the practice of physicians, who do not take the simplest medicines themselves, until a last resort, although they have been familiar with their virtue and modes of action all their lives; but as for taking patent medicines, they would almost as soon take a known poison, and many of them would rather do it, for then they would know the antidote. I do not take medicine myself nor would I advise others to take it, if the desired object can be accomplished in another way; and when administered, it is to avoid a greater damage; it is on the principle of choosing the less of two evils. Medicine should be taken in as few cases, in as small quantities, and at as long intervals as possible. I think the time is approach-ing when those will succeed best in effecting remarkable cures, who will give the least medicine, and resort more to the employment of physical expedients, external remedies, and dietetic means.

A young man applied to me, supposed by his friends, and fearing himself, that he was in the commencement of consumptive disease: he had oppression; pain in the breast; could not lie on the side for pain; rapid pulse; mother died of consumption; difficult breathing; started to ride on horseback to my office, but from weakness and pain had to return; these things had continued for some months. By taking a single pill, using a special form of exercise, at specified hours in the day time, washings and frictions at particular parts of the body, and a regulated diet, he got perfectly well within a month, and remains so to this day. This young man was killing himself by being employed twelve hours out of the twenty-four, in a singularly stooping and confined position of body; and all the syrups, and balsams and balms that could be purchased, would not have saved him from a speedy death; but a system of physical remedies did save him, by counteracting the destructive tendencies of an unnatural position and confinement. This case is given to show how much a little medicine will accomplish, when accompanied with appropriate observances, founded on the causes of the malady and on the circumstances with which the patient is surrounded.

REMARKABLE CURES.

I was once called to see a man, who had cough, hectic fever, night sweats, with great debility and emaciation. He was said to be in the hopeless stages of consumption, and had for a long time been confined to his room. A country physician was in attendance, and reported to me that he had employed the usual remedies in such a case, but without the slightest apparent benefit; on the contrary, the cough, and night sweats and debility were getting worse every day. I left a few pills of rhubarb and aloes, with special directions about diet, air, exercise, clothing, and cleanliness. In a few weeks he was able to make a full hand on a farm, and subsequently grew to be a corpulent man, and died in the south four or five years afterwards of yellow fever. Strange as it may appear, this man, in his debilitated condition, compelled to lie abed sixteen hours out of every twenty-four, was making a hearty dinner every day of fat bacon and boiled cabbage, with breakfast and supper in proportion, which gave him an incessant, dull pain at the pit of the stomach, keeping him groaning for hours every day.

A wealthy Kentucky farmer, one of those hospitable gentlemen of the olden time, whose integrity of character was without a stain, and who delighted in deeds of peace and kindliness to all about him, had what was termed a " sore toe;" it had some time before been injured accidentally in such a way as to have the end of it cut off; but it healed up and was forgotten, until after a season it became inflamed, hard and painful. A great variety of neighborly recommendations, which " couldn't do any harm, if they didn't do any good," were resorted to without benefit. A country physician was consulted; next a city practitioner, but not being able to relieve him, they advised amputation as necessary to the saving of his life. Matters were thus assuming a very serious nature, the pain could be no longer borne, and the alternative was the loss of life or the loss of the ailing member; but before submitting to an amputation, he was advised to consult my brother, Dr. Sam. Hall, of Fourth street, Cincinnati, who, having spent some time in the French Hospitals, had acquired a simplicity in treating surgical cases only to be obtained from opportunities of extensive observation, and who considered it a mark of " greater skill to save a limb than to cut it off neatly." He recommended him to take no medicine, and to submit to no operation, but to bathe it half an hour every day in simple warm water, and after each bathing, to grease it well with sweet oil. This gave prompt relief, and in a short time the troublesome member was perfectly well. How did this happen? The skin over the end of the toe had become perfectly hardened, and constant pressure on the nerves of the part, had set up a degree of irritation and pain scarcely endurable; the applications softened the part, removed the inflamation, soothed the irritation, and reduced the skin to its natural state.

A young lady had a painful affection of the throat, coming on at a regular hour every day. Every thing that could be thought of was tried to no purpose. Last of all, caustic in solution was applied daily for a month, without any effect whatever. My brother advised her among other things, to discontinue the caustic altogether, and by persevering in the use of a gargle of simple cold water, she soon reported herself to him as perfectly well.

C

The above cases are given to show that there is more to be done in the practice of medicine than to employ the knife and administer drugs: to show that by a judicious observation, and the exercise of a sound judgment, some of the most grievous ailments, and the most threatening diseases may be warded off and permanently cured, by pertinent appliances, and with almost no medicine at all. Persons have even ceased to take advice of me, because I "expected them to get well without any medicine."

I do not wish the reader to understand by what I have just said, that I do not give any medicine, for there are complications of disease which make it necessary to be given freely and often. I am only showing how much good may be done, and how much suffering saved in other ways than by swallowing physic from morning till night until a man makes an apothecaries shop of his body. If I have any theory at all, it is never to take a particle of medicine for any ailment, if it can possibly be removed in any other safe way. My object is, NOT to show how much I can do by a great "cure all" medicine, or patent apparatus, but to show how much may be sometimes done without either; to show my disapprobation of all patented contrivances and compositions for the alleviation of human suffering; and that I have no respect for their authors or for those who by trafficking in them, make themselves partakers in a crime against afflicted humanity.

PRINCIPLES OF CURE.

If I have succeeded above others in the treatment of consumptive diseases, it has arisen from the following considerations:

Practising in these diseases and in none other.

Detecting the disease in its earliest stages.

Persevering in a course of treatment in spite of repeated backsets and discouragements.

Never doing anything to weaken the patient.

Avoiding confinement to the house, even in cold weather.

Considering cough a curative process, and therefore using no measures to smother it, as all patent remedies do without exception. The cough should be got rid of gradually, by eradicating the causes of it, instead of smothering it up, as is the common practice by the use of opiates in some of their forms.

In consumption, whatever weakens, makes worse; hence I never applied a plaster and never made an issue, because these do weaken in many, very many instances, besides doing other injuries occasionally, which are not recovered from for months, if ever. Many persons have come to me who have been blistered from the chin to the pit of the stomach, when they averred that they "never could see that it did them any good; while they did suffer a great deal of inconvenience and pain from them, and seemed to get weaker every day." The strength of the patient ought to be increased from the first hour, by safe means; and this I always endeavor to do, and carefully avoid doing anything which by any possibility might weaken. It is thus that persons sometimes express surprise at "feeling stronger daily, without taking anything."

MEDDLING WITH COUGH.

An error which many persons fall into, in the treatment of consumption, is in meddling with the cough. In my larger publication, pp. 98, cases are given to show that a troublesome and long continued cough may exist, and nothing be the matter with the lungs. In all such cases, all remedies addressed to the lungs must fail; and he who in a real case of consumption, at once sets about to destroy the cough, destroys the patient. Many a person says, "If I could only get clear of this troublesome cough, I would be as well as I ever was in my life." Another will say, "there is nothing the matter with me but a little cough." a third will come in and say, "Doctor, I am not sick, and I don't want to go through a course of medicine, I only want you to give me something to cure this cough. I have a good appetite, and sleep sound when I do get to sleep; bowels regular, and I feel hearty and strong, but this cough is always pestering me; just give me some drops to take it away and I will be well as I ever was in my life." A case :—I was once called to see a very estimable lady, whose worst symptom was a most distressing cough; she complained of pains about the breast and neck and of several other things of minor importance. I told her the cough was deep seated, that it would require all her efforts to get rid of it, and that this would have to be done in a very gradual manner; that I would prevent her coughing at night, but that the cough during the day must be borne with, as it aided in bringing away the constant accumulations, otherwise, she would soon have her lungs fill up, and would suffocate. She, however, became impatient, and being remiss in following some of my directions; I ceased to prescribe for her, after seeing her four or five times. Some one was called in who had "cured several cases worse than she was in a few days." His medicine seemed to have a good effect; in a day or two the cough sensibly declined, and finally ceased altogether and with it the expectoration, and about the same time, she died. And it is thus that thousands are destroyed every year; they purchase various syrups and cough remedies, and because they moderate the cough, they think they are getting well; losing sight of the fact, that they are getting no stronger, or losing flesh, or that the dose has to be increased; and as soon as they cease taking it, the cough returns, proving conclusively that it is only a palliative, while the main disease is working its way deeper into the system.

OPINIONS OF CASES.

With these views in reference to consumptive disease, I will give a few illustrations of the correctness of my judgment in cases presenting themselves for an opinion, as many come for an opinion only; the reader will at the same time have an opportunity of seeing the character of the opinions, not only as to their correctness, but that they are plain, direct, concise, to the point, and always in writing.

An over anxious mother brought to me her daughter, aged eighteen, of great personal beauty and perfection of form: she complained of constant head ache; cold feet; great chilliness; occasional dry cough; pains through the breast; also in the left side, and sometimes in the right; quite sore there; indisposed to exercise; variable appetite; heavy pain at pit of stomach; has spit blood several times.

Opinion: "Your daughter's lungs are perfectly sound in every part of them; all her ailments, are the consequences of having nothing to do but to eat and frolic. Make her go to bed at ten and get up at five; ride four miles and back in a fast trot, canter or hard gallop before breakfast, and the same before tea; take nothing for breakfast and supper but cold water and brown bread and butter; eat nothing between meals; take a moderate dinner of what she likes best; not sleep a moment in the day time; take a fast cheerful walk of an hour after breakfast and during the afternoon: scrub the whole surface of the body for ten minutes, night and morning, with a coarse towel dipped in salt, and then sponge with cologne water; she needs no medicine, she will be well enongh in two weeks." And it was so.

570. S. U., aged 21, pulse 100. Slight wandering pains in the breast; hands cold; feet burn; dull hurting weight at stomach, which swells, and the weight of the clothes is oppressive; has spit up clogs of dark blood every morning for several weeks past; family consumptive.

Opinion: "You have no consumption; your lungs are unusually good; your disease is simply acute dyspeptia; and by correcting the deranged condition of the stomach and liver, you will get well." This man perfectly recovered in a short time.

572. W. J., aged 30, six feet high, pulse 100. Dry cough on getting up; weak in the limbs; weight and uneasiness at stomach; eye-sight impaired; hair falling off; aching in throat if talks much; voice hoarse; some difficulty in swallowing liquids, at times; difficult breathing: numbness in left side; fallen off twenty pounds; don't sleep four hours in twenty-four.

Opinion: "Yours is a disease of the stomach, liver and bowels; nothing more. There is not a better pair of lungs in the city, that work more freely and fully. You will get well if you go to the country and chop wood all day in the open air; go to bed at ten o'clock regularly, and get up the instant you wake every morning; live altogether on cold bread and butter, fresh meats, stewed, ripe fruits and cold water; swallow three teaspoons of white mustard seed, whole, three times a day, an hour before meals; chew slippery elm bark freely during the day; spit out the bark and swallow the juice; scrub the skin to redness, twice a day, over the neck, breast, sides and stomach, with a woolen flannel, dipped in salted alcohol, and you will be well enough, soon enough." In three months afterwards, he wrote me that all the above symptoms had disappeared.

K. H. G., farmer, aged 24, height, six feet and one inch. Fallen off twenty pounds; a hard cough night and morning; occasionally during the day, causing him to throw up his food; difficult breathing; loose bowels; voice hoarse for two months; throat stings when water is swallowed; tall, square, rawboned man; brought this on by going barefoot in April, to harden his constitution; thirst every forenoon; very chilly; pain between shoulder blades.

This patient brought me the written opinion, just given, of one of the most distinguished surgeons in the United States; which was as follows:—

" Oct. 2nd, 1848, 3 o'clock, P. M. Respiration 31 per minute; pulse 130; Broncophony in the upper part of each lung; respiratory murmur scarce audible on the left side of the chest; very little expansion of the left thorax during inspiration; most of the same side flat on percussion; condensation of a great part of the left lung; a degree of hypertrophy of the heart, with probable dilatation; bellows murmur in the passage of blood through the heart; defective valvular function.

Prognosis unfavorable.

The opinion I gave the father in writing was as follows.

" Your son has true consumption; the left side of the lungs is in a state of decay; a large quantity of decayed matter is still there, and the decay is progressing. One third of his lungs being hopelessly lost to him, recovery is utterly impossible; if nothing is done for him, he will probably die in two months; the best directed efforts will save him from some suffering, but cannot possibly protract his life longer than three months." He died in ten weeks.

713, M. C., September 18th. She is in the last stages of consumption; a large part of the upper portion of the left lung is utterly gone, the decay is rapidly progressing, and nothing can arrest it; her death is inevitable before the close of the year.

COD LIVER OIL.

The above opinion was given of a young woman, never married, full cheeks, and to look at her sitting at the distance of a few feet, you would not suppose any thing was the matter with her. A lady brought her to me, who was worth some sixty thousand dollars, and instead of consulting a physician in time, had been giving her cod liver oil for nearly two years, and had very recently ceased giving it. When she came to me she could not speak above her breath, no appetite, bowels loose, and costive alternately; cough night and day, daily chills, feet cold, the slightest exercise produces exhaustion; pulse one hundred and twenty, and breathing while at rest, sixty a minute; her courses had never appeared. Here was a holy human life thrown away; a young woman's existence sacrificed, from degrading penuriousness. The history of this case was shortly this; from some neglect or exposure, the courses did not appear; a physician not being consulted, a slight cough followed, wholly depending on the disordered condition of the uterine function; thousands of such cases are cured every year by judicious physicians, with very little medicine; but this wealthy woman, thinking it a case of bginning consumption, became, in order to save the expense of consulting a phy-sician, her own family adviser, and administered the above article vigorously, for two long years, until the patient was at death's door.

The blind administration of cod oil has hurried many to an untimely grave, and will destroy many more; because

The common article is absolutely unfit for use, and it is so horribly nauseous that many are utterly unable to use it, and declare they would rather die than continue to take it. When compelled to take it by superiors or from motives of economy, as the common kind is had at one or two dollars a gallon, while the light colored and pure is, up to this time, afforded at ten dollars a gallon, and is almost impossible of attainment; when, I say, persons are compelled to take it, it often brings on symptoms, worse than those sought to be removed.

Even the pure oil, made of Livers not over a day old, and gathered in January, is, in nu-merous instances, inappropriate; as in the case above, or in liver cough, &c.

When there is no fever, no irritability of pulse; when the bowels are regular, the liver healthful and digestion good, it is a valuable remedy; its value and its virtues are wholly de-pendant on its being well digested; and when this is not the case, it is only a source of in.

creased irritation and ill health. It is affirmed, also, by those who have strongly advocated its use, to produce in numerous instances spitting of blood; one of the most alarming of all symptoms, and very justly so, as it very generally ends in cough, consumption and death; in fact, it is but too often the case, as intelligent physicians very well know, that blood, spit from the mouth, coming from the lungs, even in small quantities, is the unwelcome symptom of decaying lungs; that is of consumption in its latter stages. How careful then should persons be of taking anything, without a physician's superintendance; of taking anything which, by a remote possibility, is followed by so unwelcome and fatal a symptom.

IMPOSITIONS.

I wish to give here, an additional warning, that the pale oil, sold by many druggists as the pure cod liver oil, gathered from fresh livers, taken in mid-winter, is a spurious article; being made of a mixture of sweet oil, lard oil, bromine, iodine, and other articles. The Druggists themselves are not aware, in many instances, that the article is adulterated, or rather fabricated, being imposed upon by the Eastern Dealers. The only safe plan is to take oil under the advice of a physician who is personally acquainted with the manufacturer, who himself procures, or by his agents, the fresh livers at the fisheries in the Northern Atlantic, coast of Labrador and Gut of Cansor.

Then, and only then, can you be assured of two things.

First, that you have a pure and genuine article.

Second, that it is applicable and not hurtful in your case; without these assurances, no sane man ought to use it.

Such being the circumstances connected with its employment, it is, perhaps, destined, like other good remedies, to do more harm than good; and like them, for the same reasons, to fall into disuse. I am truly glad that, hitherto, I have been able to get along without it; having been prejudiced against its trial, from four principle causes:

Its unreasonable costliness.

The almost impossibility of getting the real article.

Its inapplicability in numerous cases.

Its acknowledged hurtfulness in others, inducing diarrhœae, hæmorrhage, &c.

In the above cases, as well as in all others, I endeavor to express the convictions of my own mind at the time of the examination, either to the patient himself, or to the nearest relative or friend. I am paid to give my opinion, founded on a careful examination of each case. It can in no instance answer any ultimate good to mislead. If the lungs are not diseased, it would be cruel not to remove the heavy weight that hangs on the mind; and if they are diseased, the patient ought to be made fully aware of his situation, that he may be stimulated to use every effort possible, and that, too, without delay, for an alleviation or an entire removal of the disease. No one will make the requisite effort, if the truth be partially concealed; on the other hand, if the disease has arrived at an incurable stage, a man ought to know it; and the sooner the better; that those preparations may be made, which the present and the future call for.

FOOD,

Its DIGESTIBILITY, NUTRITIVENESS and time required for its DIGESTION.

The following table is one of very general interest and utility; a much more extensive one will be found in the *Appendix Edition*. The time required for the digestion of food, and the ease with which it is digested, do not always accord; nuts for example, and oils are more nutritious than boiled rice, yet the latter is digested in one hour, while the former require several hours. Food which is most nutritious is marked the highest; wheat, for example, is marked ninety-five, because out of one hundred parts, ninety-five, that is, 95 per cent. of it is taken up by the nutrient vessels, and applied to the nourishment, and support, and strength of the system.

The article of food most difficult of digestion, is marked one, the easiest, ten. For the table giving the time in which food is digested, the world is indebted to Dr. William Bcaumont, of St. Louis, Missouri, to whom was allowed the rare opportunity, never thus afforded to man, before or since, of looking into the stomach, while digestion was going on, seeing it with his own eyes, watch in hand; hence his statements are taken for granted by all eminent medical writers throughout the world. The orifice, which is still open, was made in the stomach of Alexis St. Martin, who is yet living, on the sixth of June, 1822, by the accidental discharge of a musket, loaded with powder and duck shot.

KIND OF FOOD.	MODE OF PREPARATION.	AMOUNT OF NUTRIMENT.	TIME OF DIGESTION.	EASE OF DIGESTION.	
			h. m.		
Almonds,	Raw,	66			
Apples,	Raw,	10	1.50	5	Sweet and mellow.
Apricots,	Raw,	26			
Barley,	Boiled,	92	2	5	
Beans,	Dry,	87	2.30	4	Boiled.
Beef,	Roasted,	26	3.30	3	Fresh, lean, rare—broiled is dig. in 3 h.
Beets,	Boiled,	15	3.45	3	
Blood,		22			
Bread,	Baked,	80	3.30	3	Warm Corn bread, is easier of digestion.
Cabbage,	Boiled,	7	4.30	2	Raw cabbage " "
Carrots,	Boiled,	10	3.15	3	
Cherries,	Raw,	25			
Chickens,	Fricasseed,	27	2.45	4	
Cod Fish,	Boiled,	21	2	5	
Cucumbers,	Raw,	2			
Eggs,	Whipped,	13	1.30	7	
Gooseberries,	Raw,	19			
Grapes,	Raw,	27			
Haddock,	Boiled,	18			
Melons,	Raw,	3			
Milk,	Raw,	7	2.15	5	Digest in 2 hours if boiled.
Mutton,	Roasted,	30	3.15	3	" 3 " broiled.
Oats,	Oat Meal,	74			
Oils,	Raw,	96	3.30	3	
Peas,	Dry,	93			
Peaches,	Raw,	20			
Pears,	Raw,	10			
Plumbs,	Raw,	29			
Pork,	Roast,	24	5.15	2	Raw or stewed, digest in 3 hours.
Potatoes,	Boiled,	13	2.30	4	Broiled or baked, " 3½ "
Rice,	Boiled,	88	1	10	
Rye,	Rye Bread,	79			
Sole,	Fried,	21			
Soup, Barley,	Boiled,		1.30	7	Meat soups digest in 3 to 5 hours.
Strawberries,	Raw,	12			
Turnips,	Boiled,	4	3.30	3	
Veal,	Fried,	25	4.30		Broiled digests in 4 hours.
Venison,	Broiled,		1.35	6	
Wheat,	In Bread,	95	3.30	3	

The condition of the bowels is a matter of the first importance in all stages of consumptive disease, more especially in the advanced stages, when they are inclined to be loose ; it often happens that consumptive persons die of loose bowels, when the lungs are sufficiently whole to have allowed them to live in comfort for years to come, could the bowels have been regulated to act but once a day.

Blackberry cordial is the most agreeable of all non-medicinal agents, in diminishing the frequent, thin and light colored passages ; to be prepared thus :—

Put the blackberries in a pot of water, boil until the juice leaves them, strain through a flannel bag; add spices, loaf sugar, cinnamon and cloves to the taste, then boil again for twelve minutes, skim, and let cool. To three quarts of this juice add one quart of the best French brandy.

TO BOIL RICE.

Take a pint of Rice, wash it well, then soak it two hours in cold water ; have ready two quarts of boiling water with a little salt in it, in a stew pan. Half an hour before you wish to use the rice, pour the water from it, in which it has been soaked, and with a table spoon shake the rice gradually into the stew pan, without stirring it ; let it boil ten minutes, then strain the liquid from the rice ; return the rice to the stew pan, and let it steam fifteen or twenty minutes, a short distance from the fire, it will then be done, and the grains will be separate ; add a *little* butter, and send it to the table.

In graver cases, it should be prepared as follows :—wash it well, then parch it brown or black like coffee, and while a pot of water with a handful of salt in it, is boiling, sprinkle in the rice, bad grains being removed, and let it boil twelve minutes by the watch, stirring it all the time ; pour off the water, cover up the vessel, place it a little distance from the fire, and when cool enough, eat it with a little butter or sugar.

The general principle as to diet, in the management of loose bowels of all kinds, is to use such articles of food as have the most nutriment, and the least waste ; hence, boiled rice alone will cure in many instances, while raw cucumbers will kill, because rice, boiled as above, has eighty-eight parts of nutriment in a hundred, and only twelve of waste, to be carried off over the the tender and inflamed surface of the bowels, while cucumbers have only two and a half parts of nutriment, and ninety-seven and a half parts of waste matter to be carried from the system. Hence the saying that *rice is binding*, whilst the most untutored know that raw cucumbers, boiled cabbage and the like, are charged with death. In times of cholera and spring diarrhœas, this table should be studied closely by every one, and all medicine most carefully avoided; even burnt brandy and loaf sugar, unless advised by a careful and experienced family physician.

It is of importance, sometimes, to have the best kind of bread. Corn bread should always be eaten warm and fresh ; wheat bread should be two days old, and cold or toasted.

Vegetable food contains, almost fully formed, the three great ingredients of the human body, viz: Fat, Bone and Muscle or flesh, and that kind of food which contains these in the largest quantity, is the most wholesome; hence, brown bread made of wheat ground and used without separating the bran from it, has one third more nutriment, and is much easier of digestion than when bolted ; that is, made into fine white flour, by having all the bran taken out of it. Professor Johnston gives the following as the amount of nutriment contained in one thousand pounds of unbolted flour and common flour.

Unbolted Flour.			Fine Flour.		
Muscular Matter	-	150 lbs.	Muscular Matter	-	130 lbs.
Bone Material	-	170 "	Bone Material	-	60 "
Fat	-	29 "	Fat	-	20 "
Total	-	348			210

That is to say, there is, in a thousand pounds of brown bread, one hundred and thirty-eight pounds of nutriment *more*, than in a thousand pounds of bread made from common white flour ; and the finer and whiter the flour, the less nutriment does it contain, and the more difficult of digestion.

Such kind of brown bread, with rice, prepared as above, roasted potatoes with plain fresh meat, not killed within six hours, well cooked, cut up in pieces not larger than a pea, and taken in moderate quantity, and not more than half a glass of fluid of any kind, constitutes one of the most easily digested and nutritious meals that can be devised for a weak stomach, especially if a moderate walk be begun in ten minutes, and continued in the cool, pure air, for half an hour or longer.

As to apples and fruits in general, they are good at all times if eaten in the early part of the day, at regular meal time; they should be perfectly ripe, without a spot or blemish of any kind, and should be eaten raw or roasted, but not between meals, nor after the middle of the day.

The above table is often referred to in my prescriptions, and it should be carefully preserved.

A person in good health will extract nutriment from the following articles in the proportions named.

100 lbs. of Lentils have	94 lbs of Nutriment.		
" Peas	- 93	Meat (average)	35 lbs.
" Beans	- 92	Potatoes -	25
" Rice -	88	Beets -	14
" Wheat	- 85	Carrots -	12
" Barley	83	Cabbage -	7
" Rye	- 80	Greens -	6
" Bread (average)	80	Cucumbers -	2

TERMS OF TREATMENT.

To many persons, this is an item of considerable importance, and a degree of relief will be experienced in their having some definite statements made on the subject.

Many desire to have my opinion only, as to what is the matter with them, without reference to treatment ; for such on opinion, which is always expressed in writing, as on page *Thirty-five* the charge is - - - - TEN DOLLARS.

For advice by letter, *per month*, remedies *not* included - - TEN DOLLARS.

Do. at my office *per week*, remedies included - - TEN DOLLARS.

Remedies per box, when necessary, lasting from 1 to 2 months - TEN DOLLARS.

I do not give advice in any case, for a less amount than Twenty Dollars ; for, being given in print and in writing, it is so full, that in numerous instances, persons have got entirely well with but one set of directions. See *Appendix Edition.*

The *average* cost of cases which have come under my care, has not exceeded *thirty-five* dollars. If I did not limit the time, the great majority of persons would not follow out my prescription vigorously, and I should soon have a larger correspondence than could possibly be attended to.

Should persons need advice beyond the first two months, they can pay me at the the rate of ten dollars a month, or five dollars for each visit made, or letter written to me after that time ; this liberty does not extend beyond one year from the first prescription.

For further particulars, see printed card, furnished to all who apply.

In NEW ORLEANS, my office opens November tenth, at 127 Canal Street, corner of Baronne Street, and closes May fifteenth.

In CINCINNATI, it opens during the last week in May, and closes on the first day of November, of each year, on FOURTH STREET, South side, third door east of Vine.

My Book is sold by J. D. Thorpe, No. 12 West Fourth Street, Cincinnati, and by J. B. Steele, No. 14 Camp Street, New Orleans. Inquire for Dr. Hall's *Appendix Edition,* which contains the treatment of some of the most remarkable cases of cure which have come under my care. Price, One Dollar ; Mail Edition, or full bound.

APPENDIX EDITION.

DISCONNECTED OBSERVATIONS, TABLES, &c.

Among the greatest medical men of modern times, are those who feel conscious of the uncertain and deceptive character of all means hitherto practiced, for ascertaining the true condition of the lungs, in cases of real or supposed consumption.

Doctors Graves and Stokes say :

"It is scarcely credible how far Laryngial obstruction tends to mask all the stethescopic phenomena, even in case of extensive pulmonary disease. Large excavations and numerous tubercles have been found in the lungs, on dissection, when, during life, no unequivocal evidence of this state of the lungs had been derived from the use of the stethescope, and we have already seen how uncertain general symptoms and percussion both, are."

At the Bellevue Hospital, Dec. 11, 1848, a woman entered with a cough, feeble and emaciated, and gradually failed until death. On examining the body, the lungs contained numerous tubercles, and a part of the upper portion of one lung had decayed away ; there were tubercular ulcers in the kidneys, ureter, and bladder; the whole system was tuberculated, the urine was always loaded with pus, and yet examination previous to her death, "did not detect any decided evidence of the presence of tubercles in the lungs ;" exhibiting another instance of the extent to which tubercular disease may proceed, without causing any characteristic constitutional disease." N. Y. Jour. Med., No. XXXVI.

The Edinburg Medico-Chirurgical Review, admitting the uncertainties of perussion, ausculation and stethescopy, says of the mode which I have adopted for ascertaining the condition of the lungs:

"The deficiency of the lungs for holding the healthful amount of air needed for the wants of the system being ascertained, the inference that disease exists somewhere, seems established with a painful certainty. The lungs, we conceive, will be found in fault in the vast majority of instances, and as there is no one of their diseases which is apt to have so long a period of latency, and afterwards to be so obscure and doubtful in its progress as consumption often is, it is especially on this disease that this new method is calculated to throw light. Subsequent experience, in several cases, verified the melancholy anticipations of the author, *where consumption had not previously been suspected.* Farther experience of the reliance to be placed upon this method of examination will, in all probability, constitute the measurement of the lungs, a valuable diagnostic in the hands of medical men. Our best ground of hope of combatting consumption successfully, is found in our being enabled to recognise it at its commencement, with certainty, so that we may attack it early and act against it with earnestness. Now this new method promises to give us this advantage, and we shall watch its future use in diagnosis with much interest and hopefulness."

Andral says : " The stethescope does not reveal consumption with certainty, without other signs. And Dr. Lathan admits that the best auscultators have been led to a wrong prognostic by it.

Trousseau gives a case of "a baker, aged 18; came to Hotel D'ieu ; had often spit up mouthfuls of red blood, with daily chills, for five months ; had general emaciation, pale skin, sunken eyes, sharp features, a bright blush on the cheeks, intense pain in the throat, altered voice, expectoration of lumps of yellow matter, night sweats, and small rapid pulse ; he lingered in this way four months, and the lungs, after death, *presented no alteration.*"

He gives another case, of Mr. L., of Dunkirk, whose lungs were found, after death, to be " loaded with tubercles, in their whole extent ;" and while he was alive, the complete loss of voice, the large quantity of pure yellow matter expectorated, hectic fever, diarrhœa, emaciation, night sweats, all concurred in demonstrating it to be a clear case of consumption; a fact which *we could not establish* by stethescopic signs. It was exactly the case with M. Prevot, a relation of Dr. Honore; he was

D

affected with consumption of the throat and lungs, in the last stages, and neither percussion nor auscultation enabled us to recognise the presence of consumptive disease."

Here, then, are acknowledgments from the most learned physicians of modern times, that there are no certain means known, by which consumption could be positively designated in all cases, *even when in its last stages,* when almost an entire lung was rendered useless by disease or by decay; but the mode which I have adopted for ascertaining the true condition of the lungs, is so precise and minute that, according to the admission of the London Lancet, if one cubic inch of the lungs is diseased, it is detected by a deficit of forty-seven inches in the amount of air which the lungs ought to have contained; and this last amount is capable of being measured, down to one cubic inch; consequently, if one forty-seventh part of an inch of the lungs is lost by decay, or is otherwise rendered useless, it is immediately and easily detected; and, furthermore, what must be a source of the highest satisfaction, as the patient is getting well, this deficiency is constantly decreasing, as is evidenced by actual and simple measurement, from week to week.

That a man should measure his improvement in getting well of consumption, though novel to many, can be more easily imagined than the application of the Sonometer, which has recently been exhibited in London, by which the capacity of the ear is precisely and accurately measured, as regards its exact appreciation of sound; and the most simple and uninitiated may decide what progress has been made towards a cure of deafness. See London Lancet of October 11th, 1849. Nor is it at all as complicated as the mode of measuring muscular strength, recently proposed by M. Emiles du Boys-Redmond, who communicated, through Humboldt, to the Academy of Science, at Paris, a description of the following experiment, that establishes the fact of the electrical influence of the human system. Fix to the two extremities of a sensitive galvanometre two strips of platinum—plunge these slips into two tumblers of salt water, and then introduce into the tumblers the corresponding fingers of each hand. Let them remain until the fluctuations of the needle cease. Then contract the muscle of one arm by an effort of the will, and a deviation of the needle will instantly indicate a contrary current of electricity in that arm. The amount of deviation depends upon the *muscular development.*

When I first began to devote my whole attention to the treatment and cure of consumption, my medical associates prophesied a certain failure and inevitable starvation; I was fully aware of the fact that many considered it disreputable, and very likely there are some who still think it so. Such persons are, however, behind the times, and are ignorant of the world they live in. There is scarcely a respectable medical quarterly published, that does not contain one or more articles written by men of note in the medical world, going much farther in their expressions of belief in the curative nature of consumption of the lungs—going much farther, I say, than I have ever done: they advocate recovery from the very last stages of the disease, while I have spoken of its certain cure, only in its first stages; in all my publications I have directed my chief attention to the instruction of the people as to the symptoms of consumption in its very first beginnings; the importance of then making an effort for its removal, and giving assurance of its hopelessness in its advanced stages. So that while I was at one time several years in advance of the age, I am now behind it. Then, I was, perhaps, the only living, regular graduated physician who practiced, exclusively and literally so, in consumptive disease, not merely in America, but, as far as I know, in the world; but to-day, while I write, many have followed; extensive hospitals have been erected, and others are in progress, for the purpose of treating consumptive patients exclusively.

I lately visited the Infirmary, built in London, for persons having consumption; the subscription list for its erection, having been headed by the Royal family and numbers of the nobility. Since that time, a hospital has been built at Brompton, for the same purpose, and it has been recently " proposed in London, to found an establishment in Madeira, for the reception, at a very moderate expense, of consumptive patients in the middle classes of life."

" The People's Journal, for July, of the present year, one of the most popular European publications, has an interesting article in relation to the Consumption Hospital, founded at Brompton, five years ago; and few institutions have risen so rapidly; it has a long list of noble and wealthy subscribers, with the Queen and most of the Royal family at its head. 'As death has abundantly proved the mortality of the disease, so, paradoxical as it may seem, death also supplies us with evidence that the chief structural lesions of Consumption, *tubercles in the lungs, are not necessarily fatal.* The writer of these lines can state, from his own observation, (which has not been limited, and is confirmed by that of others,) that, in the lungs of nearly one half of the adult persons examined after death from other diseases, and even from accidents, a few tubercles, or some unequivocal traces of them, are to be found. In these cases, the seeds of the malady were present, but were dormant, waiting for circumstances capable of exciting them into activity, and if such circumstances did not occur, the tubercles gradually dwindled away, or were in a state of comparatively harmless quiescence. This fact, supported by others, too technical to be adduced here, goes far to prove an important proposition, that consumptive disease is fatal by its degree, rather than by its kind; and the smaller degrees of the disease, if withdrawn from the circumstances favorable to its increase, may be retarded, arrested, or even permanently cured. There are few practitioners of experience who cannot narrate cases of supposed Consumption which, after exhibiting during months and even years, undoubted symptoms of the disease, have astonished all by their subsequent, more or less, complete recovery. Cautious medical men have concluded themselves mistaken, and that the disease was not truly tuberculous; but, in these days, when the detection and distinction of diseases is brought to a perfection bordering on certainty, the conclusion that recoveries do take place from limited degrees of tubercles of the lungs, is admitted by the best authorities, and is in exact accordance with the above mentioned results of cadaveric inspection. Consider properly, and you will be ready to admit the truth of what has been already established by experience, that *Consumption may be often prevented, arrested, or retarded by opportune aid.* On this point we know that many medical men are utterly incredulous, and stigmatize others who are less so, in no measured terms; but, with the present rapid improvements in all the departments of medical knowledge, there is less ground for such incredulity than there was for that which opposed and ridiculed Jenner in his advocacy of vacination as the preventive of small pox.'"

THE CURABILITY OF PHTHISIS.

"The writings of Laennec, Andral, Cruveillier, Stokes, Williams, and others, prove that many cases of pulmonary phthisis (consumption) have, contrary to all expectation, recovered; and that, at a subsequent period, death having occurred from some other malady, the lungs have been found puckered and cicatrized from the healing of the tubercular cavern. The more recent researches of Roget and Boudet, in Paris, and J. Hughes Bennet, in Edinburgh, have shown, from the indiscriminate examination in large hospitals, that puckerings, cicatrices, cretaceous concretions, and other evidences of former tubercle in the lungs, occur in at least one-third of all the individuals who die after the age of forty in this climate. Facts, therefore, indicate that so far is pulmonary tubercle from being necessarily fatal, it is spontaneously cured by nature in a *vast number of cases,* and that in not a few this is accomplished, even when large ulcers have been formed in the lungs, and all those symptoms present which are considered evidences of so called consumption.

The curability of (understanding by that term, recovery from) consumption, is a matter, therefore, which no longer admits of a dispute. It is a fact as certain as the curability of pneumonia, or the union of a fracture, and, like the latter, is susceptible of demonstration by means of well-preserved preparations. [*Monthly (British Medical) Journal, October,* 1847.]"

Such is the testimony of the most popular Medical Journals in the world, in reference to the curable nature of consumptive diseases, and in commendation of those who attempt its cure, despite of opposition in high places and in low, where the educated few and the ignorant many unite in one common prejudice; the one party too ignorant to examine, the other too self-sufficient, too lazy, or too proud.

Dr. Gillersdet, of Sweden, in a large work on consumption, says that, "cases certainly do occur where every symptom of the disease exists, but the patients, nevertheless, recover their original health," and, with Reynaud, he affirms that "caverns in the lungs may heal in two different ways; in one case, the parenchyma surrounding the cavern becomes indurated; in the other, it shrinks, draws together and forms a long, firm, white cicatrix. The fibrous bands which surround the pulmonary parenchyma, compress the tissue of the lungs by contracting, and thus materially assist the healing of the excavations.

Dr. Addison, of Guy's Hospital, London, says that " the natural cure of an excavation in the lungs, consists in the formation of a more or less permanent living membrane, the true cicatrix of such ulcers."

Dr. Hancock's testimony is, that " Rush, Portal, and the most judicious physicians have constantly regarded consumption as a disease of the constitution, and in the times of Moreton, Sydenham and others, it was not regarded as an incurable malady."

Rokitansky and Engel, in their magnificent work on morbid anatomy, state that the following diseases or conditions are *curative of consumption; Goitre or swelled neck, Rickets, Arterial Disease, Venosity, Cyanosis, Enlargement of the Heart, Pigeon Breast,* lateral curvature of the spine, compression from pleuritic exudation, pregnancy, all kinds of abdominal enlargements, any considerable developement of the abdomen and its viscera, persons suffering from a protracted cold in the head, from Asthma, and bronchial dilatation, were known in Laenneacs time to enjoy an immunity from consumptive disease, or have had it arrested in its progress, permanently, by their antagonism.

All these things promote the cure of Consumption in its latter stages, by their mechanical action ; that is, by compressing the lungs, any existing cavity has the matter contained in it, pressed out, and thus the way is prepared for a healing process, just as the matter must be necessarily pressed out of a common boil, before it can heal, as the commonest observer must know ; and as the cough aids in bringing that matter away, to suppress that cough by opiates and cough medicines, is the most certain method of killing the patient. The rational mode of cure is to cut off the supply of that matter, instead of preventing its removal by quelling the cough ; instead of doing this last, I have even found it necessary to use every means to increase the cough and the case R. B., given on page 49, got well, and I consider it one of the most remarkable cases of recovery in my practice.

The mechanical effects of the different conditions above named, tend to the cure of Consumption in another way; the matter of a cavity is not only pressed out, but the sides of the cavity are pressed together, and at once begin to heal, just as a cut across the arm will heal if the sides are kept pressed together, and never can heal if those sides are held asunder ; and to empty a cavity, keep its sides together, and raise to, and maintain the general system at the highest point of health, is my main object in every case.

Marshall Hall says :—

" In some cases of Laryngitis, the patient cannot snuff up the nostrils so as to draw in the sides of the nose, the *Alae Nasi.*

Difficulty in swallowing is a frequent symptom of ulceration about the voice making organs.

Laryngal cough often occurs in fits, with hoarseness and difficulty in speaking, sometimes inducing vomiting.

Tracheal cough is lower, less violent, and without hoarseness.

Bronchial cough is lower still.

Sometimes a disorder of the stomach and digestive organs induces cough, leads to copious secretion of mucus, and finally to actual disease.

The expectoration of four or five tablespoons of pure red blood, without previous symptoms or muscular effort, is very alarming, being usually the first symptom of tubercles in the lungs.

Consumption of the bowels is the most insidious of all those diseases which may be considered as necessarily and progressively fatal in the course of four, five or six years ; its prominent symptoms are cold feet and hands, frequent pulse, and slow but steadily progressive emaciation, great sensibility to the slightest unexpected exposure, as opening of a door, and the patient usually creeps to the fire."

Tubercular Consumption never comes on in any other way than by a gradual decrease in the action of the lungs ; and this symptom precedes every other; it precedes even the regular hacking cough. I measure the action of the lungs, and the very moment I perceive a settled decrease from the natural, healthful measurement, of a few inches, I pronounce that man in danger, because he is just taking on Consumption. However free he may be of cough, yet if his measurement is decreased with a uniformly rapid pulse, the very first bad cold he takes, will leave a cough that ends only in the grave.

If there be a material decrease of lung action, with a pulse steadily above its natural standard of ten or twenty beats, I treat that man as a consumptive, though he may never have noticed a cough, may eat heartily, have sound sleep and regular bowels ; for in all such cases, an experienced auscultator will discover the prolonged expiration of present tubercles, and any slight cause will develope the hateful " hack."

If, then, a person comes to me with a slight cough, pulse natural and the lungs in full operation, giving their utmost healthy measurement, I pronounce that man utterly free from consumptive disease, in spite of cough, matter expectoration, night sweats and spitting blood ; and a little medicine, judiciously administered, proves the correctness of the opinion.

Consumptive diseases advance with advancing civilization ; the old stock, who lived in log cabins, and on plain substantial food, are still among us, and in some instances have outlived their generation ; their children have grown up, dwindled and died, even before their prime, while they live on, to mourn their memories. In many cases, not one is left to perpetuate the family name—not one, out of a large circle of connexions. The principal causes of this melancholy fact are universal neglect of physical education, and ignorance of the general physiological laws of the human system. Many presume on their good constitution ; some are thoughtless, unobservant, reckless ; others have too much ambition ; overstrain themselves ; work too much ; think too much ; worry themselves into disease, because every thing does not go on precisely as they could desire it ; habits of over-eating, idleness and late and hearty suppers, feather beds ; straps ; suspenders ; braces and tight dressing ; sleeping in close, small rooms. These causes are in constant operation, sap away the vitals, and by unseen degrees, leave but a wreck behind, of what was once a noble constitution.

It is impossible to benefit a consumptive patient, except in proportion as the liver, stomach, and bowels are kept in constant healthful action; because, unless this is the case, proper nutriment is not derived from the food, the blood becomes poor, and the patient weakens. I wish that all physicians would take note of this.

Nothing gives any substantial benefit to a consumptive patient, unless it have a tendency to nourish the system, or enable it to draw nourishment from what is taken into the stomach.

The great mischief in consumption is weakness; and the only way to remove that weakness, is to add nourishment, for that only imparts real strength. Many medicines give strength, but this is the difference ; the same amount of nourishment, always imparts the same quantity of strength, and the general effect is a decided improvement ; while the same amount of deceptive medicine, soon loses its effect, and must be increased in frequency or quantity, hence it is always advised to *increase the dose* in one of these respects. Whenever I do give *medicines* in this disease, the invariable rule is to diminish the dose, sooner or later, but never to increase it.

It is well expressed by Ranking, that " in the successful treatment of consumptive disease, debilitated digestion must be excited, nutrition regulated, secretions reestablished, the lymphatic system stimulated, and the organic nervous system modified ;" and it is the wildest absurdity to suppose that any one agent, or routine practice, can accomplish these diversified requisitions, and duly regulate the necessary apportionments ; even to determine how much of this, or that, or the other, is demanded in any particular case, requires the exercise of the most mature judgment and the most practised skill; making it almost akin to insanity for any one, even a physician, to attempt these things for himself, in his own person, on his own responsibility.

" In consumption, an *effort* in breathing is early visible, and its effect seen in a movement of the sides of the nose ; it is also early observed to be short on any exercise, especially on going up stairs ; and finally there is constant labor and shortness of breathing."

I propose, in the following pages, to give some cases which have come under my care, without naming the disease, or the reasons for the treatment, or the mode of action of the remedies given ; I wish simply

To state the symptoms,

To name the remedies employed,

To give the result,

and allow the reader to form his own opinions, to draw his own conclusions, and to frame such theories as may suit himself. It is not my intention to offer certificates or letters of recommendation, I do not think any respectable physician would submit to such a mode of extending his practice. I will simply state facts and let them take care of themselves.

2. J. N. J., carpenter, aged 26, having a wife and one child. He was building a bridge at Louisville, Kentucky. was very much exposed to wind and water, and took a bad cold, which lingering for some time, he called in a physician, who prescribed for several months, and the patient still getting weaker and worse, he advised him to return to his family, that he was in consumption and he could not do anything for him. He did so, and two neighboring physicians were called in, one of whom had practised medicine in Pittsburgh for *thirty years*. After treating his case for several months without any apparent benefit, the man in the meantime having got so weak that he was only able to sit up in an arm chair while the bed was made up, they abandoned it as hopeless, and I was sent for.

On entering the room I found a number of the neighbors present, the wife weeping by his side, the patient himself was asleep, lying on his back, his mouth open, his eyes half closed, showing the whites; the face was very pale except some redness in the cheeks. He woke up with a wildness of expression in his eyes, and for a while spoke incoherently. His pulse was ninety-five, his breathing short and rapid, bad taste in the mouth, pains between the shoulder blades behind, along the breast bone, through the breast and at the pit of the stomach, some little pain in the side, headache, bowels costive, great nervousness with difficult breathing, cough very troublesome exciting nausea and vomiting, had frequent night sweats and spitting of blood a year ago, had great weakness and was much emaciated, had a daily morning chill and a craving appetite. He was taken two years before with weakness and spitting of blood, occasioned by lifting and hard work in making bridges.

I ordered from one to three pills a day, each containing two and a half grains of socotorine aloes, one grain and a quarter of colocynth, and one quarter of a grain of sulphate of iron.

To take in a teaspoon of syrup of sarsaparilla one and a quarter grains of bromide of potassium and half a grain of bromide of iron, three times a day, about an hour before meals.

For breakfast, light or brown bread two or three days old, and butter good and fresh, with *one* cup of coffee or tea, half of it boiled milk, or which is better, a glass of cold water.

For supper the same.

To eat not a particle of anything between meals, and

For Dinner, to take what best agreed with him of plain, substantial, nourishing food; preferring fresh beef to other meats, roasted or broiled, and cut up in pea-sized pieces before it is put into the mouth, to be eaten with good, strong mustard or catsup; to take but one kind of meat at a meal, with cold, light bread and but two kinds of vegetables, giving the preference to boiled turnips, tomatos, roasted Irish potatoes, boiled rice, sago, tapioca, *and nothing else*.

I ordered an ammoniated liniment for the breast, to have the room well ventilated, and to use an inhaling tube three times a day before meals.

I heard nothing of this man for four days, not knowing whether he was dead or alive; his physician having stated he would give me a thousand dollars if I would raise him up, I had some desire to succeed.

On the fourth day I received a note, saying: "night sweats gone, feel very well this morning, pulse ninety, am walking about." Whether this was written by himself or by his direction, I do not now recollect.

On the fifteenth day from the time I first saw him he rode to my office, four miles, and returned without any inconvenience.

At a later date he sent me word that he believed he had caught cold by loading a wagon with corn in the corn-field; this was about the first of November. He continued to improve, and was dismissed. The next summer he called to see me, having gained in flesh some fifty pounds.

At the end of four years he called at my office on his way to the South, to make a fortune, being, to all appearance, a well man.

16. Miss E. D., She came to my office October 26th, 1843, dark hair, black eyes, elegantly formed, in the dawn of life. Her face was pale and thin, pulse 85, yellow tongue, bitter taste, head ache, pain in the small of the back, cold feet and hands generally, bowels costive, some nervousness, a very troublesome dry cough, expectoted matter streaked with blood. She was taken with a bad cough and had been ailing for some months; her parents and friends considered her case a hopeless one; they had no expectation of her recovery. She got well, and what was better, got married, and better still, is the healthful mother of three or four fine children. I saw her but once.

The treatment was, in addition to the other case, to ride several hours on horseback every day; as soon as she rose every morning to put both her feet at once in cold water ankle deep, for a minute or two, rubbing them well with the hands all the time they were in the water, then wipe them with a towel, then hold them to the fire until they were perfectly dry and warm in every part, rubbing them with the hands all the time, and just before going to bed at night to heat them by the fire, rubbing them with the hands for at least a quarter of an hour, until they were dry and hot, and then to get into bed as quick as possible, having extra cover from the knees downwards.

26. N. M., merchant, aged thirty, pulse 96, bitter taste in the mouth, white dry tongue, pain between the shoulder blades behind, sometimes so severe as not to be able to sleep, pain under the edge of the ribs on the left side, flying pains through the breast, irregular bowels, difficult breathing at night, and on going up stairs or up a hill, drenching night sweats, a hacking cough, tough phlegm, had fallen off one sixth of his whole weight, was taken seven months before with a very bad cold and cough, brought on by exposure to a variable atmosphere and an open window: breathing very quick, complains most of shortness of breath.

This gentleman got well in due time, and remains so to this day; has a family and is a successful merchant in one of the handsomest and most flourishing cities in the west.

With the general treatment and remedies named in the first case, I ordered common vegetable pills so as to have one or two passages from the bowels daily, no more, no less.

30. W. J. M., a tall handsome maiden in her "teens," pulse 84, bad taste, frequent head ache, a constant soreness between the shoulders for six years, pains in the breast and side, a very troublesome cough, father died of consumption, and several relations on the mother's side. This estimable young lady got well in due time; has since married, and remains well at the end of six years.

39. N. F., grocer, aged 22, height six feet one inch; bad taste, pain in the head sometimes, and in the centre of the right breast, great deal of general chilliness, especially along the back, costive bowels, restless sleep, nervousness, difficult breathing, cough troublesome after lying down, three or four hours hard cough at night, not so easy as in the day time, expectoration yellow, with white frothy, bubbly stuff, as much as a quarter of a pint in twenty-four hours, considerable night sweats; taken with a bad cold by sleeping on a flat boat. He soon got well under the general treatment, and five years afterwards he called at my office weighing one hundred and fifty pounds, pulse 72, to all appearance a healthy, hearty man.

41. F. D. W., miner from Dubuque, aged 26, pulse 100, mouth dry, and has a bad taste, tongue white and dry, pain and weakness in the small of the back, a dull, heavy pain in the head, sometimes for a week or two at a time, can't stoop over or stir quick, pain across the upper part of the breast, also under the ribs on the left side, a falling away, fainting feeling at pit of stomach, and weakness, if fasts long, feet cold at night and always dry and husky, has taken a great deal of medicine, pills, sarsaparilla, &c. difficult breathing when he goes to bed, and coughs, followed by a feeling of fulness at left of breast bone, cough is very troublesome, most so when he gets up in the morning, excites nausea occasionally, expectoration of a lightish cast, streaked with yellow; was taken a year ago with a cough by going to a fire; father and sister died of consumption several years ago; has the most inveterate, spiteful cough I have ever known. The instant he enters a room he begins to cough and coughs on without intermission from five minutes to half an hour, leaving him al-

most exhausted, the same kind of cough is excited if he laughs or attempts to whistle, or engages in common conversation; had a great straining three years ago, something gave way across the breast in lifting a weight, his greatest inconvenience is, when sitting long has a pain round under the ribs, fails about the stomach when he exercises much, if he stands still he fails about the back. Under the same general treatment mentioned above, he was at the end of a month no better; a change, however, eventually took place, and at the end of some months he wrote to a merchant in New Orleans that he could whistle as long, laugh as loud, work as hard and lift as much as any man in the neighborhood, and as far as I know, remains well to this day.

53· W. B., aged fifty—brought to my office from a private hospital, being expected to die every day from an affection of the lungs; he was borne into the room by two strong men from a carriage at the door; great general chilliness, expectorating yellow matter, with binding across the breast and a feeling of rawness along the breast bone; some emaciation. Perhaps it may give a more correct impression as to the condition of this gentleman by stating that his friends considered it doubtful whether he could live longer than a few days.

I dieted him as in the first case; caused the whole surface of the body to be well and often scrubbed with coarse cloths dipped in salt water; one quarter of a grain of Sulphate of Morphia every night at bed-time; the bowels were regulated by Cook's pills from day to day; the inhaling tube was freely used; for a troublesome and steady pain in the side, I ordered persevering frictions and the application of stimulating liniment; these things were kept up steadily, and at the end of one week he walked out, and shortly afterwards was able to walk several miles a day; his cough became less and less, and finally disappeared, his sleep and appetite returned, and now at the end of six years he has not the slightest remnant of any of his former ailments, and with a pulse of seventy, and a respiration of eighteen a minute, he has as sound a pair of lungs as any man of his age, with better general health than he has known for more than twenty years.

505. E. H., A young lady of seventeen, a planter's daughter, was taken with spitting of blood while in apparent perfect health, a sister and brother had died of unmitigated Consumption, both of them had walked about the streets until within a day of their death, and the afflicted mother was in the greatest grief and alarm; the young lady herself was lying on the bed pale and frightened; to see her on the street no one could have imagined her otherwise than in robust health; the cheeks were full, all the muscles well developed, and there was no one appearance of any disease whatever; but on a near view at the bed side, the actual condition was very different; the cheeks were mushy and of a bloated paleness, the muscles of the arms and limbs, instead of having the firmness and solidity of health, were compressible, yielding and flabby to a remarkable extent. Some ten months before, she had gone to a fourth of July party and got wet while menstruation was in progress, the courses were checked and had never again appeared. A very distinguished surgeon was in attendance at the same time; on examination he thought she would follow her brother and sister. I thought if the courses could be restored, she would recover and gave directions accordingly.

I ordered the diet of the first case. The same attention to the feet with the additional item of wearing constantly in each stocking foot half a teaspoon each of ground mustard and cayenne pepper, to ride from ten to twenty miles every day, rain or shine, on a trotting horse among the mountains for six months; to prevent the constipation of the bowels by the free use of ripe fruits of all kinds, to embrace every opportunity of running and romping in the woods with girls of her own age, to swing herself by the limbs of trees; every morning on getting up, to wash the neck, chest, and arms in cold water, the colder the better, to continue this washing for at least eight or ten minutes, then with the mouth full of cold water, take a coarse towel, dipped in cold water, or have a pair of gloves or mittens made of coarse tow linen, and dipping them in water, begin at the feet and rub upwards fast and hard, as far as can be reached in every direction and along the spine, and while rubbing over the breast lay one hand on the other and rub as hard as you can, so as not to break the skin; continue this rubbing until the whole skin is tender or red, then rub on lightly with the hand a table-spoon or two of cologne water, all over the body every morning, but to the neck and chest only at night; let the previous rubbing be such that when the cologne water is applied, there shall be considerable smarting, and after the morning rubbing, dress quickly and take a run or rapid walk or horseback ride for an hour, but never go out of your chamber of a morning for exercise, especially in foggy weather, without chewing a crust of bread or common cracker.

The friends and family of this young lady considered it under the circumstances a matter of life and death; the directions given were put in requisition and observed to the utmost letter, and with the most fortunate of all results, a perfect restoration to all the healthful functions of the body, which continue up to now, the second year. I did not advise a particle of medicine.

517. June 10th. R. B., aged 28; merchant, six feet high, wanting half an inch, slender made, had weighed one hundred and sixty pounds, now weighed one hundred and eighteen, pulse 100 in a minute, had a constant pain in the breast, could not cough without pain; he was very sorely afflicted with piles, exhausting night sweats, great weakness, jaws were flat, thin and sunken, the eyes were large, round and blue, thin, lank, light hair; he would stagger out of my office with sheer debility; he was a Scotchman; I never knew a man of more honorable bearing; he was possessed of singular mildness of character; under the most acute suffering, when calamity was piled upon calamity, he seemed to have an increasing acquiesence in the Almighty's will, and yet was resolute in his endeavors for a restoration to health. His night sweats became perfectly drenching, and nothing could control them. There seemed to be a large collection of matter in the hinder part of the lungs, and the accumulation became so great at length, that the pain was almost insupportable day and night. The piles were so bad as to prevent his sitting down without pain, and for the same reason the pain in his breast would not allow him to lie down in any natural position; his lungs contained 172 cubic inches of air instead of 258, and altogether the case was discouragingly hopeless. I told him that it was essential to his safety to get clear of the large accumulation of matter in the lungs, and that I knew no way of accomplishing that but by increasing his cough, in the hope that it would enable him to throw it up freely. As most consumptive persons are inclined to cough more in some positions than in others, I directed him to observe what position in his case inclined him to cough most, and to maintain that position for a great part of the time; but this did not avail; fomentations of strong liniment, the skin rubbed and cloths saturated in hartshorn and alcohol bound on to the parts seemed to do no good, while the daily accumulations were going on, he could get no rest at night; I was afraid for his mind, as want of sleep is a frequent cause of insanity. As a last resort, I administered freely quinine and elixir vitriol to have a constringing effect on the system. I was induced to do this, from having persons to tell me after taking it for several days, that their cough was worse. I took means at the same time for relieving the piles; his strength improved a little, and the pain decreased from freer expectoration. It was now the middle of July and the city was insufferably hot and dusty, and although he was scarce able to walk across the street without great fatigue, I advised him at once to go to Canada, believing that a fresher, purer and cooler air at a country residence would do him more good than all medicine. I told him I thought he would certainly die if he remained in the city—and although his recovery was extremely doubtful under any circumstances, I believed that such a change of locality presented the highest probability of recovery. He did not think he would be able to reach the lakes, but undertook the journey. He reached the Falls of Niagara in safety; but on his arrival a horse fractured one of his leg bones by a kick; and to show his own views of his condition, I here give a few words from a letter dated July 23d: "I hope the Lord will enable me to spend the few days I shall linger out here in making a perfect preparation for that place where our state is irreversibly and forever fixed."

Six months afterwards, I met a gentleman in New Orleans, in crossing a street, and thinking him the brother of this patient, I stopped him to inquire, although he was walking rapidly; but it was my patient himself, just returned in a ship from New York. He had no symptoms of any disease, and seemed in every respect well, his lungs having nearly regained their natural capacity; they never could do that altogether, because they had in part decayed away.

In all my practice, I never had a more remarkable case of recovery than this; by the mercantile house in New Orleans through which he was introduced to me it was regarded and spoken of as "almost miraculous." As far as I know, he remains well to this day. He corresponded with me while he was in Canada, and kept up rigorously the general plan of treatment, which consisted in

D2

Regulating the bowels by means of a prescribed diet—
Several hours exercise in the open air daily, rain or shine. As his limb, however, was injured, he could take none for a while, except on horseback.

He was to take cold bread and butter only, with weak tea or coffee for breakfast and supper, to eat what he wanted at dinner, to eat nothing between meals; to take before each meal three quarters of a grain of sulphate of quinine; to use an inhaler, to use extensive and frequent friction to the whole surface of the body, and then apply a stimulating liniment- The part affected with piles to be washed night and morning with cold water, the feet to be heated by the fire every night, the last thing on going to bed, and to be put in cold water every morning, both in at once, ancle deep, for a minute or two only.

In reference to the fears which some people have of going out of doors, and their inability to take exercise, I will only give as a confirmation of my views an extract of a letter from this gentleman a few days after he left me; the reader bearing in mind that when he left me, he himself feared he would not live to reach Canada via the rail-road.

"I take the liberty of addressing you a few lines just to inform you how I got along since I left you three days ago at Cincinnati. I am happy to inform you that, notwithstanding the fatigue I experienced during the journey, having had to sit up all night in the cars from Urbana to Sandusky, yet I have stood it beyond my most sanguine expectations." And he continued to improve from that day forward until his recovery.

AN IMPORTANT CHAPTER.

The air we breathe is essential to life; if a man is wholly deprived of it for three minutes his death is certain.

It is essential to life because it is the last process of digestion. We sustain life by eating, the essence of all the food we take is turned into blood, but the last step, and the one by which it becomes blood, is its coming in contact with the air; this union takes place in the lungs.

In proportion as the blood is pure we all have perfect health. There can be no disease in a body where there is no impure blood; and the only object to be accomplished in curing any disease, is to purify the blood and promote its proper circulation; indeed, if pure, it is in effect self circulating.

No blood, then, can be made without contact with pure air, and it is by means of the lungs that this contact is brought about; see page twenty-one of my large fifth edition, 8vo. 1849.

The two essential processes of life, then, are
The proper breathing of pure air;
The proper circulation of pure blood.

And as it is the air which turns the essence of food into new blood, and constantly renovates and purifies that which is already made, two things are essential to health and life; that the lungs should always work well, and that they should always have a full supply of pure air; and in proportion as they do not work fully, or in proportion as the air they respire is impure; in such proportion always, and under all circumstances, will the blood become impure and disease and death in due time invade the human frame, gradually and in all its parts. This is the essence of consumption, beginning as it does at the very foundation of life, and impairing the whole structure; not one single part, not one single atom escaping the slow withering influence; how justly called "a decline," for if every fibre of the human body is not at every instant receiving a fresh supply of pure blood, that instant that fibre begins to decay and die, as certainly as a fish begins to gasp and die the instant it is thrown upon the shore.

The respiration and circulation are so entirely dependant upon one another, that when one is impaired the other begins immediately to feel its influence, and the same as to restoration to health.

Thus it is that in consumption the circulation and respiration are always deranged, the man breathes oftener and the pulse beats faster in proportion as he is nearing the grave. In consumption the breathing and the pulse are more frequent than they ought to be, and are more easily excited in every hour of the twenty-four.

The pulse is excited because the breathing is rapid, and the breathing is rapid because the lungs do not take in enough air at a time to satisfy the thirst of the blood for air. Beyond all question, then, the very first step toward actual consumptive disease, is the lungs habitually not taking in as much air as the system requires for purifying the blood, and to detect this decrease in its smallest, almost inappreciable beginnings, is to detect consumption in a stage so early that it is as easily arrested and cured as any other chronic disease, and even easier, because no internal medicine is required; and this is the very thing I most certainly do; because I know how much air a man's lungs ought to take in if they were in a whole condition and in full healthful operation. For example; Capt. B. came to me in New Orleans on the fifteenth of March for an opinion of his case; his lungs should have contained two hundred and forty six cubic inches of air, whereas they contained but one hundred and ninety two, with a weak pulse of one hundred and a respiration of thirty to the minute. I told him that he had true consumption, that his lungs were in a state of decay, and if not arrested, he would certainly die within a few months. He called on the twenty-second and said that he had been conversing with an old physician in good health, an old associate of his, for whom he had a very high respect; this physician had at one time been very ill, as all supposed with consumption; however, by the use of medicinal remedies he recovered. In detailing his symptoms, the Captain thought that they bore a remarkable similarity to his own, and became fully possessed with the idea that his, also, was a liver affection, and that a course of blue mass would cure him. I represented to him that he was mistaken, and as an inducement, offered to give him advice and remedies without charge; but he declined them, saying he would follow his own course, and if he did not get better, he would call and see me in two months, as he was compelled to go to Pittsburgh.

In my note book, vol. 6, case, 636, I find the following remarks.

Thursday, March 22nd.—This case has lost confidence in my treatment; that is, my opinion with him is below par.

2. He will die this summer, or, at least, before next winter, because he will not follow my treatment.

3. Because he believes it is his liver solely, and will act accordingly.

4. He will die, because he averages eighty cubic inches of air less than he ought to have at each full inspiration. His pulse is still one hundred, and his cough I consider a terrible one, and there is an alarming thinness of flesh.

I never saw him afterwards, he died on the twenty-fifth of June following.

There is another item in this case worthy of remark. When he came into my office on the fifteenth of March he was weak and emaciated, and coughed badly; he had a severe pain in the right side, no sleep, no appetite, tongue dry and rough; he had an exhausted and haggard expression of countenance, and was greatly dispirited. With some minor directions, I gave him to take at bed-time a pill made of four grains of calomel, one grain of ipecac. and one-tenth of a grain of tartar emetic, made up with distilled water. He returned in two days, saying, as he entered the door, "I could not have believed that so great a change could have taken place in so short a time." He continued to improve for the week he was under my care, and the action of his lungs had been increased from one hundred and ninety-two to two hundred and twenty. His cough had diminished, slept well, without any kind of annodyne, appetite good, and in other respects was doing well. But in spite of all this improvement, and his own acknowledgement, he became possessed of an unfortunate idea, that the liver and not the lungs, was at fault, and perished, the victim of a mistaken opinion. Doubtless, this man would have continued under my care, especially under so marked an improvement, if I had fallen in with his views, told him that I had made a mistake, that it was his liver, and that I would treat him accordingly. But in dealing with a man's life, I cannot, I will not yield to his prejudices or ways of thinking, even for the chance of saving his life. I give the convictions of my own mind; I am paid to give my opinion; I have done it hitherto, and intend, in all cases, to do it hereafter; and persons who cannot abide by that opinion had better stay away. It is dishonorable to deceive a man on the verge of the grave; to say nothing of a higher consideration, the morality of it.

In order to let the reader see how beautifully, as I think, my system of treatment operates, in connection with the subject at the head of this article, I will give a case or two illustrating this point; that persons under my treatment for consumption measure less air than they ought to do, fast pulse, fast breathing, &c.; but, provided their cases are curable, they do from time to time measure more air, the pulse falls, the breathing is less rapid, the strength improves and flesh increases.

FREQUENCY OF BREATHING DIMINISHED.

August 2nd.—A tall, spare, raw-boned man, six feet one inch high, with black hair and eyes, aged 49, weighed once 180 lbs, now 135, only. " I caught cold," said he, "two years ago by getting wet, it settled on the breast; was in excellent health until that time; have taken a great quantity of patent medicines since, but have got steadily worse; I now sometimes spit up in a day half-a-pint of thin, pure, yellow, ragged matter; I cough a great deal, sometimes two hours before I go to sleep, then I wake up about midnight and have another spell of coughing, and another as soon as I get up and stir about a little."

He was greatly dejected, had three spells of spitting of blood, within two years, mixed with matter; his cough was most distressing, coming on about every two hours during the night, so that when he gets up in the morning he feels weak, exhausted and wretched. I fear that too many of my readers can fully appreciate the meaning of his statement by sad experience. The opinion I gave is as follows; verbatim. "You have consumption. One-tenth of the lungs have decayed away, therefore, you can never get entirely well again. No medicine known to me will do you any good, but an injury; anything that will speedily stop your cough will kill you before Spring; except by accident, you will not die soon, but by proper exercise, avoidance of fatigue, &c., you may live for years to come."

I gave him the usual advice, and in a week or ten days he returned, to all appearance worse than he was before, more feeble; he now could not sleep at all, except by snatches of a few minutes at a time; he said he could hear the clock strike every hour of the night, and that toward morning he was drenched with sweat. He insisted upon it, that without speedy and very marked relief he would die soon; that he could not stand it; he could get no sleep; his fits of coughing were so frequent and so long continued, that when they were over he sank down perfectly exhausted, they left him feeling as if he would rather die than continue in such a horrible state of endurance.

I told this man that I saw nothing to change my views of his case, that he certainly was not going to die, and that all that was required in addition to what he was already doing, was to go home, and at bed time every night, to wrap a wet sheet around his breast, and if it got dry in the night to wet it again, and take it off in the morning. I gave such directions in addition as would keep him from taking cold. He said he was afraid it would kill him; yet he was willing to try anything that would do him any good.

In a week he returned. He said the first morning after using the wet sheet around his breast, it smelled so badly that he was obliged to fling it away from him; this smell gradually diminished, and finally disappeared. He could sleep some, and his cough was not so bad.

At the end of two months, viz Oct. 4, I find the following entry. "Walked four miles this morning, and feel stronger and better than when I first started, appetite good, strength keeps gaining, bowels regular; my disease has changed, I cough only by spells, and do not cough much at night when I cough and spit up freely in the day-time. The tickling and soreness at the little hollow place at the bottom of the neck in front is not so bad now, and when I sleep it does me good; breast is well enough now; sometimes I do not cough once in half-a-day. . As his bowels, sleep, appetite were all good, no sweating, almost no cough, all soreness around the middle from coughing and straining had disappeared, was getting stronger and gaining flesh every day, he wanted to know if he needed any farther attendance."

August 2,—32 respirations in a minute.
Sept. 26,—28   do.
Oct.   4,—20   do.

This case is to show, that as a man gets well of breast complaint, the breathing is slower and slower, until it gets down to the natural standard, which is generally from 16 to 20 in a minute.

ALTERATION OF THE PULSE.

As persons are recovering from consumptive disease, the breathing is not only slower, indicating that the lungs are in a condition to take in enough air for the wants of the system, that is, that their measurement has been increased under the treatment until it has reached about its natural standard, but the pulse at the same time gradually diminishes in frequency. The case I shall now give also shows that as a man is getting well, while the pulse becomes less and less rapid, the capacity of the lungs to contain air increases.

656. W. B., a merchant from Kentucky, aged 33, pulse 96, taking in at a full breath 170 cubic inches of air, instead of 254, that is, one third of his lungs were useless to him, either because they were hopelessly decayed away, or collapsed, infiltrated with mucus, &c. The instrument which I use for measuring to the fraction of one cubic inch, how much air a man's lungs hold at a full inspiration, does not indicate in any way the cause of inoperative lungs; it only shows the fact that they are inoperative, and the physician must determine by auscultation and other general symptoms, whether the lungs are decayed away or whether they are merely engorged, collapsed, infiltrated or the like ; and this is a matter of vital importance, for if they are gone, their restoration is hopeless; if, however, they are within a man, and are merely rendered useless by the latter named class of causes, these causes of inaction may be removed ; so that with the instrument which I employ for measuring the capacity of the lungs for common air, a man must be a finished auscultator, and must be most thoroughly acquainted with the whole catalogue of symptoms of diseases to which the human frame is liable. But before I give the opinion rendered in this man's case, I will detail some of his other prominent symptoms.

He was a tall, spare bachelor, with a white dry tongue, a great deal of pain in the small of the back for the last two years, constant pain in the breast, and frequent ill feeling between the shoulder blades behind ; he had a great deal of general chilliness, (and no wonder when he had lost the use of one third of his lungs,) burning feet and hands in the afternoon, costive bowels, linen generally damp from night sweats, a dry hacking cough night and day, always on getting up in the morning ; has spit blood at different times for four years past ; at one time he spit up clear red blood every day for three weeks ; the cough was his greatest inconvenience. He thinks his ailment was brought on by having had the measles some years ago, they did not come out well. Complains of being always chilly, and looks as if he were almost frozen ; he has fallen off, from his best weight, twenty-seven pounds. With these symptoms, I gave him the following opinion :

"Your general constitution is much impaired by long standing disease, and your lungs have suffered much in consequence, so much so, that a large portion of them are useless to you ; they are inoperative, inactive, and do not answer the purposes of life. *A part of your lungs have decayed, but that was some time ago ;* that decay is not progressing at this time ; your lungs are not decaying now; but they are in such a weak condition, that you are liable at any time, by any debilitating sickness, or by a succession of bad colds, to be thrown into a rapid decline. It is my opinion that your lungs can be restored to their full action, and your health placed on a good foundation."

The reader will please notice the words above in italics. After he had read my opinion, he said to me for the first time, that about five years ago he went to the south for his health, and the physicians told him that he was in the last stages of consumption ; shortly after a running sore appeared not far from the socket of the thigh bone ; he at once began to recover and got well.

When he first came to me, his pulse was 95, and his lung capacity 170 ; on the 27th of August his pulse was as low as 90, and his capacity 186 ; on the 24th of August, just seventeen days after, his pulse was 80, and his capacity 230. I have not seen him since, (some six weeks ago,) but I have no doubt I shall find a continued improvement, and a dimunition of six or eight for the pulse, and an increase of 24 cubic inches of lung capacity for air, would restore him to his healthy standard. The reader will here note the correctness of my opinion, not only in telling him that his lungs had been previously diseased; but that he could get well again, notwithstanding night sweats, constant chilliness, and an incessant cough. Not only his pulse and breathing improved, but he had a correspondent increase of strength, flesh and appetite, no sweating, no blood, bowels regular, and he did not complain of cough at all. It may be interesting to the reader to know what I did to produce these changes.

I required him to be out of doors five or six hours every day, rain or shine, on horseback, or walking up and down hill with his mouth shut, to run 50 or 60 yards and back three times a day with all his might, with his mouth full of water, increasing the distance a yard or two every day, until he could run two hundred yards and back, and continue at this until he could perform it without much weariness or fatigue. I gave him a liniment to apply night and morning to his breast, back and shoulders, or wherever else there was any unnatural feeling; made thus: one sixth Tincture of African Cayenne, one sixth Tincture of Alum, one sixth Tincture, or rather saturated solution of common salt, one sixth Tincture of Gum Camphor, one sixth Tincture of Hartshorn, one sixth ninety-two per cent. Spirits of Wine.

I ordered one pill every ten days of four grains of Calomel, one grain of Ipecac., and one twelfth of a grain of Tartar Emetic, and for six days after each pill to take one hour before each meal, in a wine glass of water, one grain of Sulphate of Quinine, and two drops of Elixir Vitriol. I gave also an inhaling tube, and diet as follows:

BREAKFAST.—Cold light, or hot corn bread and butter, one Irish potatoe roasted, *or* one or two roasted ripe and perfect apples, *or* one or two soft boiled or whipped fresh eggs, with one cup of weak tea or coffee, or which is much better, one glass of pure cold water.

FOR SUPPER.—Cold bread and butter; with ONE cup of weak tea or coffee, or which is very much better, ONE glass of common cold water.

FOR DINNER.—Eat what you want and as much as you want of plain, substantial, nourishing food, prefering roasted or broiled fresh meats, moderately done; cut it up in pieces no larger than a pea; do not eat more than one kind of meat at a meal, nor more than two kinds of vegetables; let all desserts alone, and drink nothing but ONE glass of cold water.

Do not sleep a moment in the day time, nor eat a particle of anything between meals; go to bed regularly at nine o'clock, and never remain in bed longer than eight hours at farthest.

TAKE NOTICE.—I do not wish the reader to imagine that I cure every body that comes to me; that I never lose a patient, or that I have so many patients on hand, that it is with great difficulty I can find time to attend to them at my office, or to answer their letters if they are away. I have never yet had so many but that I could find ample time to attend to more, and I am losing cases every few weeks, because necessarily, persons often come to me in the very last stages, and although I tell them there is no chance, that they must in all probability die; still they oftentimes insist that I shall at least do all I can for them, that even if I cannot save life, I may save from suffering, or add a few days or weeks or months to their existence.

I will now give a few of these cases to show that as life declines, that as the lungs are decaying or rotting away, their capacity for holding air diminishes day by day and inch by inch, until the closing scene. Thus to be able to measure from week to week how fast one is dying, is a process of very great but melancholy interest, showing how *literally* true is the popular phrase as applied to a consumptive, "*he is dying by inches,*" for every week and day and hour he is losing his lungs by the inch, and this is susceptible of the most satisfactory and convincing measurement.

349. vol. 3. A. M. Y., tall, slim man, aged 32, nearly six feet high; came to me August 14. Pain between the shoulders, weak breast, hectic fever in the afternoon, spits up several teaspoons of yellow matter every day, costive, bad cough, unrefreshing sleep, constant pain in the breast, pulse 100, lungs hold 168 cubic inches of air, instead of 254, a deficiency of nearly one-third.

August 14th,—pulse 100, breathing 18, lung capacity 168.
Oct. 15th,—pulse 90, breathing 17, lung capacity 184.
Oct. 23d,—pulse 80, breathing 14, lung capacity 192.

Here was a steady, gradual, admirable improvement, and he felt that he was getting well. Being a very close man, he thought he would obtain some of my remedies and dispense with the cost of advice. I did not see him again until the 8th of December following, a period of near seven weeks. During this interval, he injured himself by over-exertion and exposure to the mud and rain on the levee at New Orleans in November, and not feeling free to come to me, (having been remiss in using the remedies I gave him, under the conviction that he was getting well,) he applied to an eminent surgeon; but not getting better, and becoming alarmed, he called on me again.

December 8th, pulse 112, breathing 22, lung capacity 160. These three symptoms together with increased emaciation and unmistaken auscultatory signs, compelled me to tell his brother that his lungs were rapidly decaying, that there was no chance for life and that he would not live three weeks, although he was walking about the streets. He died in sixteen days, December 24th.

With cases like these, I cannot but think, and feel convinced that my mode of ascertaining and treating the diseased condition of the lungs is reduced to a perfect system, as admirably simple as it is eminently successful.

DESPERATE CASES.

I do not wish the reader to believe that I am infallible. I have sometimes been mistaken; I have frequent occasion to tell my patients this. Occasionally, persons come to me who appear to be in so hopeless a condition, that I have scarcely thought worth while to take notes of their case, except in very general expressions of their condition when they first came. Yet, some how or other, these people have most unaccountably got well, or so near so as not to require further medicine or medical attendance. A case:

677. D. C. P. A lady in middle life entered my office from a carriage at the door, so exhausted when she came in, that she was compelled to lie at full length on the sofa, with a cushion and pillow under her head. After resting some time, her pulse was 110, and breathing thirty times in a minute; conversation tired her very much, so I questioned her husband. "Has been complaining and doctoring for the liver three years, has had five children, with several miscarriages; but for several weeeks past has been complaining, and generally getting worse, until she is now just moving about, lying down a great deal, and for the last day or two lying down most of the time, her back and left side hurting her so; her medical attendant has been sent for three times, but has not come, as (so reported) he can do nothing more for her. She has exhausting fever coming on regularly every day, with drenching and debilitating night sweats, most distressing and exhausting cough all night, spitting up large mouthfuls of heavy yellow matter, no appetite whatever, and bowels bound up. The cough is so distressing, that she can scarcely sleep at all; a deathly chill comes on every morning about five o'clock, and at that time the cough is terrible; she has lost forty pounds of flesh."

At the bottom of the above description in my note book, I find as follows: "Hopeless, cannot live but a very few weeks." I told her husband that I could not promise anything, that cases of the kind generally died in from three to thirty days, and if she did not die in that time, she would get well. I told a gentleman, a near neighbor of her's, who felt interested to inquire about her, that she could live but a short time.

Two or three days after she first came to me, her husband called upon me in considerable alarm, as he thought her to be in a dying condition.

I name these things to show how low she was to all appearance.

Within five weeks this lady walked to my office without special fatigue, a distance of half a mile up and down hill, of a cold windy day. Pulse 68, regular, strong, and full, breathing 24, no cough at night, none at all at any time worth naming, appetite very good, bowels regular, no pain, no night sweats, no fevers.

In ten days more she called again, breathing 20, pulse 76, and the capacity of her lungs for holding air very near that of health, not needing farther medical advice. Here was a case that I considered hopeless, believed by the patient herself, her husband, her physician and her neighbors to be one in the very last stages of consumption, and yet she got well.

Two days ago she came to my office, having walked the distance with a child nine months old in her arms, about which she wished to consult me. She seemed herself in excellent health, stating that she weighed one hundred and forty-five pounds; at the time she came to me her reported weight was one hundred pounds, whether from conjecture or actual weight I do not know. She stated also that during the last week she had done the cooking and washing of the whole family, consisting of nine persons, besides nursing her infant a great part of the time, as it was barely expected to live.

This patient was too weak at her first visit to allow me to examine her by the new method, and I was obliged to form an opinion from the old mode of examination, auscultation &c., and from her remarkable and rapid recovery and restoration to her full flesh in the space of two months, I feel certain that her's was more a case of liver abcess than of lung disease.

Two important lessons may be learned from this interesting case:

First, That no case ought to be given up to die without a strenuous effort to save, however forbiding the symptoms may be.

Second, That I am sometimes mistaken.

I do not give the treatment in this case, because I did not keep a note of it at the time, and it would only be by guess; a thing which is not done in any of these pages.

CHILD BEARING.

Some of my patients, whom I have never seen, having ceased to bear children, have placed themselves under my care, have recovered their health and borne children again. Consumptive persons continue to bear children until their health has declined to a very low standard, finally it is so low, that reproduction ceases; but when the health is restored the power of reproduction returns at once.

510. C. B. E. complains of emaciation, sore throat, loss of voice, dry cough, difficult breathing, constant sore pains in the breast, very acute in the right side, daily chill, hectic fever, cold along the back, cold feet, &c., having ceased to bear children for some years. I advised a course very similar to that on page 48. She recovered her health, and became a mother in 18 months, and as far as I know, her good health still continues. Previous to seeking my advice, she had traveled over half the world and consulted physicians in three quarters of the globe, with nothing more than a temporary advantage.

An English lady, several years married, without children, consulted me for a throat affection. She had been under the care of an eminent physician, who thought he could cure her in a week or two, but getting no better, but rather worse, she came to me; the pain was so severe sometimes, running up from the throat toward the right ear, that it compelled her "*to cry out.*" I found the tonsil ulcerated, and her general health very much impaired. I cut out the tonsil, applied the nitrate of silver some twenty times, and with a gargle of alum and red pepper her throat got entirely well; her general health was regulated by cold bathing, frictions, out-door exercise, and blue pill. Twelve months afterwards she called upon me in New Orleans, on her way to visit her kindred in England, happy in the prospect of a child in two or three months.

There is another case, somewhat similar, in the wife of a clergyman in one of the northern counties; see also page 118 of my larger edition, 1848.

UNSEEN CASES.

The following cases are given to show that persons afflicted with serious and complicated ailments, may be successfully treated by correspondence, without ever having been seen by me. The case given on the paper cover of these pages is one in point. The first case under the preceding head is another. The following letter as to symptoms and treatment is from a Southern lawyer whom I have never seen. Having prescribed for him, I had altogether forgotten him, until the following was received, the first after I had sent him my prescriptions.

June 6, 1849.

DEAR SIR:—I began to act according to your advice about the first week in May. I have been obliged, occasionally, to omit most things for a few days at a time, when absent from home. But I have generally adhered to your directions; and I am happy to state that I have been amply paid for all trouble and all crosses of inclination; I am now in better health than I have been for five years, I feel confident that in a month or two more I shall be perfectly well. I have now no cough at all, some soreness yet remains in the breast, but it is much lessened by the use of the liniment I have only applied the liniment twice a day; I have generally applied it to the breast only, having no soreness in the throat, but only a gathering of mucus, I did not apply the liniment to the throat. It appears from the directions for using it that it is intended to remove soreness and other irregular feelings; now I should like to know whether I must use the liniment on the neck to remove the evident inflammation of the throat when that inflammation is not evidenced by soreness? The tincture of myrrh benefits my throat some, and the elm bark a great deal; but if there is anything else that can aid these agents in their work I should like to know it. My voice is far less affected, in a bad way, from speaking than before, and in the course of time I have no doubt these things alone would effect a cure. I desire to know, mainly, whether the liniment must be used on the throat as often as it is used on the breast?

My inward fevers are less frequent than they were, and less weakening. The Sunday night pill operates very powerfully; besides operating greatly on the bowels, it produces sickness to such a degree as sometimes to unfit me for business. Once I forgot the pill on Sunday and took it the next night. I have but one more pill to take to make five; please instruct me what to do next in regard to the pills.

I am now using the tube 25 minutes; I shall begin to use it 30 minutes in a few days. Let me know how to use it after the 30 minutes term expires.

You do not require me to wash all over every morning, but I have done this regularly since I began under your prescription. In washing, or rather in rubbing my breast, I have undesignedly abraded the skin, this makes the liniment cause much smarting—probably no other ill effect ensues.

If I should get fully restored to health, there are many of my friends whom I shall prevail on to try your treatment. They not being as far gone as I was, can't be induced to try the experiment now; though my decided improvement begins to raise in them some faith. I am obliged to get well even under the present prescription; but if there is anything good that you can add, please let me have it. Even now I feel that I am your debtor beyond estimate. Yours truly.

A month later I received another letter advising me of his continued improvement, and having heard nothing since, I presume he is entirely restored. His mother and two sisters had died of throat and lung affections.

CLERGYMEN.

It has been in my power to restore quite a number of clergymen who had abandoned their vocation.

618. N. M. P., aged 35. Sister died of Consumption. Has a regular morning cough, spits blood and yellow matter, costive, has piles, complains of Dyspepsia and a general decline, voice cracked and uneven, soreness in breast, a pricking and heavy aching in the throat, inconvenience in swallowing, breathing sometimes oppressed, palpitation of the heart, expectoration of clear red blood, lost twenty pounds of flesh, had taken several bottles of wild cherry balsam. He says in his first letter. "I have no reasonable doubt of having the disease in some of its forms, which has arisen in part in a hereditary taint."

I advised myrrh gargles, a mercurial pill once a week, friction to the skin, and a stimulating liniment; to abandon tobacco in all its forms, and four or five hours daily exposure to fresh air, with the usual method of strengthening the lungs. He got well in a short time.

628. B. R. J., aged 33, applied by letter Jan. 26. I give several letters of this gentleman in full, as an instructive lesson to clergymen generally; it is the history of thousands of them who ruin their constitutions in their efforts to get into the ministry, and when they get there are fit for nothing, are worse that useless, because they have no health; yet they take charge of congregations and find that it is a physical impossibility to perform all their duties, and the result is, the church is uncared for, families are unvisited, the proper instruction of the children of the church is neglected, and they grow up ignorant of its doctrines and careless of its interests; while the sick and poor have to be their own comforters; nor is this all, a diseased body gives a diseased mind, and a diseased theology is the inevitable result, full of gloom and despondency and horrors, instead of being lighted up with hope and joy and gladness and forbearance and love. Many a shower of fire and brimstone has

E

dispepsia for its sire. The greeting of a minister is a grunt or groan. The presidents and professors of theological seminaries in the United States, by their negligence of the health of the sons of the church, by the burdens which they impose and the exactions they make have made a fearful entry on the debtor's side of the page; they may indeed cram a vast quantum of superfine theology into the heads of these young men; but it is all at the expense of a rufned constitution, in which they themselves have sown the seeds of death.

Jan. 16, 1849.

DEAR SIR:—I have had a throat affection for some time, and it is the object of this communication to give you some account of my case. Before doing this, it may be proper to give you the outlines of my history for several years past. I would preface this narration by remarking, that my mother (my father was drowned when I was small,) is now sixty years old. My grand-parents lived to be much older, and I think none of them died of Consumption or an affection of the throat.

I was a farmer until I was eighteen, when I had such a strong constitution that I thought nothing could injure me. During the Spring of 1834, I commenced in Winnsborough, to obtain a more liberal education. This sudden change from the farm to the academy affected me so that I soon moved to the country where I could have a better opportunity for exercise. During my literary course of six years I had several attacks of fever and bowel complaint. Sometimes, too, after sitting long in one position, my breast would pain me. When I graduated I was so much reduced that it took a year to recruit my health. The only symptom which I had, of which I have any recollection, was debility. While in the theological seminary I again became so weak that I could scarcely walk. My abdomen and lower part of my breast became swollen, and too sore to be touched. My appetite was changeable.

I was told by my physician that I had the dyspepsia; was directed to take regular exercise on horseback, to be particular in my diet, to moderate in studying; in a word, to be temperate in every respect. I tried to follow the prescription and was soon well and hearty.

I am still predisposed to the same disease. Four years ago I became a minister of the gospel in the Presbyterian church, and located in York, where I remained until a month or two ago.

I was often warned that my loud speaking and great exertion in preaching would break me down, but I heeded not; for my principle of action always has been, whatsoever my hand found to do, to do it with my might. Hence it was no uncommon thing for me to be so much exhausted after preaching that I could scarcely ride home. I, however, apprehended no injurious consequences until about the first of last year, when my attention was arrested by an uneasiness in my throat, and a hoarseness after preaching.

During last Spring I read your pamphlet on the nature, causes, and symptoms of the diseases of the throat, and told a physician that I believed l had what you called laryngitis. He persuaded me otherwise, and said I was like he was, when he commenced to read medicine, for he imagined he had symptoms of almost every disease about which he read; I, however, thought otherwise. Even by this time I was feeble and emaciated. I had, for several months, been accustomed to preach in the evening during the week, and ride home several miles through the night air. This I found was injurious to my throat, and, therefore, quit it. During last September I preached two or three days in succession, and I was told my discourses were unusually long, loud, and animated. I was much exhausted, and felt an unusual hoarseness and uneasiness in the region of my throat. A few days after I attempted to make an address, and having spoken about ten minutes, I had to stop, owing to the pain it gave me; it was a peculiar drawing indescribable pain, as I thought, in the larynx. This was not only painful, but my whole system was prostrated with debility. By resting, however, a few days, the pain ceased and I was considerably refreshed. My physician now advised me to cease preaching for a few months; and said, if I did so I would be entirely well. This advice I found it was difficult to follow ; I had several appointments out; and when I went to tell the people that I could not fill them, I was constrained to make a few remarks, until my throat would admonish me by pain that I had said enough. Thus I tried to preach and tried to quit preaching for near three months. After preaching there would be for several days an uneasy sensation in the upper part of my throat; but after resting a few days this would cease, and I would have no inconvenience in any way until I would use my vocal organs again, without intermission, for several minutes. It is true, conversation affected me after a while, but not so soon as continuous speaking. I at last concluded to follow the advice of my physician; and to spend the time in traveling.

I have now concluded that rest alone is not sufficient for my recovery. I have been resting, so far as preaching is concerned, (and I avoid conversation as much as possible,) for about two months, and yet, I grow worse. For several weeks the uneasy drawing, or, perhaps, I might say, a gnawing sensation in the upper part of my throat has been without cessation. The larynx seems to be the part affected; on pressing it to one side there is a pricking sensation, and I often feel the same sensation without any apparent cause. I have long had a feeling as if I wished to get something out of the back of my mouth; hence, I am often hawking, sometimes bringing up a white sticky matter, but oftener nothing at all. I have constantly a disposition to clear my throat and swallow, a difficulty in breathing, which increases. I have repeatedly, just as I got to sleep, been startled up as though I was about to suffocate. I can scarcely sleep without a high pillow; but I have always been accustomed to such. For some time I have had a constant soreness in my throat; I have used nothing for it but pepper tea, which was first recommended to me for my throat, and which I have used with no apparent benefit, other than it enables me to cough up matter more easily. I cough only occasionally; more generally in the morning and at night. I am considerably emaciated and weak; and seem to become more and more so. Apart from my throat, I have no pain, only occasionally, in my breast. My appetite has, generally, been good; and bowels regular. At night I am somewhat restless, and my sleep unrefreshing. Some nights I have sweat a little, caused, as I thought, by pepper tea, which I drank. My voice has never seemed to be affected much; and, yet, reading aloud, or exercising my vocal powers in any way for a few minutes causes pain in the larynx.   Respectfully, &c.

A note came with the above, desiring an opinion of the case, and to know if a visit to me was essential. I sent the opinion, saying he need not come. In reply he writes, February 16. "You seem to think that I am in a more dangerous condition than I can persuade myself that I am in. I suppose I gave you rather a colored description of my case; the circumstances in which I was placed, were well calculated to induce me to do so."

In a few days, however, he writes again, "When I last wrote to you, I could not persuade myself that I was as bad as you seemed to think I was; but I now fear that your judgment was only too true; but I am not alarmed, and I think I am prepared for the worst. I have followed your directions in every particular, except I have not as yet ceased to speak above a whisper, though from the effect speaking has had on me for some days, it is probable I may soon be compelled to obey you in this respect also, and I will make my arrangements to do so. My throat usually feels easy in the morning until I commence talking, and for a few days past, I can scarcely speak a word without more or less pain; my vocal organs seem to be sore and unwilling to act, it requires an effort to speak. I expectorate every day several spoonfuls of a white, sticky matter, it is now more stiff and less abundant; my nose discharges still more; my feet are very cold, abdomen swollen, and I am sore at the pit of the stomach, with aching in the breast if I sit long. I have a dry, hacking cough night and morning. My throat, which all along has given more uneasiness than anything else, only grows worse, it sometimes feels dry, at others as if a fish bone was sticking in it; the disposition to swallow is not as constant as it was; I am weaker than before, and have fallen off several pounds; a little walking increases my pulse to above a hundred."

This was certainly not an encouraging letter after having been under my care two weeks; but as he had followed my directions in part only, the fault was his own. A month later he writes, "I have been doing so well, that I did not think it necessary to write to you. People tell me I look better, and I feel better, am stouter, sleep sound, appetite good. I did not cease talking loud as you advised, but I feel so much better, that I think I might soon go to preaching again. A few weeks since I had the pleasure of meeting with my old friend and class mate Rev. Mr. L. S., who has been under your treatment, and is so much improved, that he has located north of this, and is engaged in preaching." The gentleman referred to had ceased preaching for sometime before he applied to me.

Before dismissing this case I will refer to his previous letters, making merely extracts, to show more fully the nature of his affection.

Feb. 6.

DR. HALL—In a previous letter you remarked, "A sermon of half an hour's length, which is as long as any sermon ought to be, would not injure, but might be of service, if spoken in a conversational tone." From this I judge you think that I am still attempting to preach; but I have not attempted to preach for nearly four months, and I preached very little previous to that time. If you suppose me able to p half an hour you are mistaken; I might hold out once or twice, but I candidly each lieve that a persistence in doing so would deprive me of speech; for the less I talk, the better I feel. In the mornings my throat feels easy and I have no unpleasant sensations until after I commence talking. Speaking or reading aloud for ten or fifteen minutes causes a drawing, indescribable pain in the upper part of the throat; if I persist, the pain is increased, and not only so, a faint or sick feeling is caused in the stomach, and soon the whole system becomes prostrated; therefore I have given up preaching and teaching also, altogether.

I must state one fact in reference to the physicians here. I consulted no one whether I should apply to you or not. I acted for myself, and supposed I had a right to apply to any one I chose, and no one had a right to say a word against it; but I was mistaken. Since it has been known that I placed myself under your treatment, a great noise has been made about it. Much astonishment has been expressed that I should have acted so strangely. Insinuations have been thrown out in reference to your mode of treatment. Every influence has been exerted to induce me to lose my confidence in you. It is even with difficulty that I can get physicians to give me medicines according to your prescriptions."

After a long interval, I have received within a few days a letter from this gentleman, he had "returned to teaching and preaching without any perceptible injury to myself. As an evidence that my health is pretty good, I will state an accident which occurred to me several weeks ago. As I rode to a swamp my horse laid down in water about waist deep. I mounted again and rode about two miles before exchanging my clothes. I would not have jumped into the water for any consideration, and yet I received no injury of which I am conscious. I would notice *only one symptom*, my urine sometime ago was somewhat colored in the morning, from this I suppose I have some inward fever."

As a great many patients have been sent to me by physicians in different parts of the country, I am induced to think that the opposition of a few arises from a misapprehension of the nature of my practice supposing

⸱ That I am not a regular bred physician.
That I refuse to tell what remediess I use.
That I set myself up as a curer of confirmed Consumption.

None of these things can be said truthfully. As to the last item, see the first page of this book; as to the first, see the last page of the cover, and last paragraph; as to the second, I here give a letter from among others of a similar character, received by me from a respectable practitioner in the south, of many years standing.

February 2d.

Dr. Hall—DEAR SIR :—I have been anxiously expecting a letter from you in answer to one I wrote you about the 11th ult. I wished to know your mode of determining Consumption by measurement. I put Miss Mary L——n on the treatment you advised, about ten days since; visited her yesterday, met her riding out; her complexion looked healthy; says she is better; coughs less, sleeps well, with the exception of one night when she caught a croupy cold by sitting late with company, with a door and window open; voice still impaired, but not as much; the fauces bore a natural appearance."

A fortnight later he writes :

⸱ "Your kind favors of January 26th and of February 7th have been received—the former the day after I wrote you my last.

The pleasure I take in reading your communications, the confidence I have in your practice, and your request to hear from my patient occasionally, is my apology at present for writing to you.

I visited Miss A. H. last Friday—I found her improving somewhat; coughs less, pulse 10 beats less per minute, a little more appearance of the menses, sleeps well without the aid of morphine, expectoration is mucous, and not much of that, but most in the morning. I had put her on the following treatment: Pills, to be taken only about the periodical returns of the menses, made of Camphor, Quinine and Ext. Belladonna. As a tonic Iod. Ferri and Comp. Liq. Iod., with Bitters made of wild cherry and Holland Gin, together with a strict injunction to learn by heart and to go by all your directions. I gave her a vial of your Naphtha mixture to try every other week alternately with the Iodide.

I have a great curiosity to see your instrument for lung measurement. How much would one cost me? It will be out of my power to visit your city this winter for many reasons. I started there in December last, but made my arrangements at Vicksburg, and on my return met with one of your former patients, who had in his possession a valvular tube whose object is to expand the lungs, &c. From this and your description of the instrument, I have a pretty correct idea of its operation; but there is nothing like seeing. With great respect, I remain your friend, &c.

Another physician, April 17th, writes: If you should not change your prescription after receiving my last letter, and continue the medicine now used, it would be well to give me the recipe for your Bitters and Diarrhœa mixture as requested in my last, and I can either fill it or get it done in Columbus." Two weeks later he writes: " I have found the bowel mixture to do well where I have used it, and thank you for the recipe." And I will only add, there is nothing in my practice which I have refused to communicate, or which I desire to be kept secret, for no honorable physician would confine to his own bosom the knowledge of a remedy which his brethren might use to advantage in the alleviation of human suffering.

CLERGYMAN—THROAT-AIL.

A young clergymen of considerable promise applied to me for a throat affection, with general constitutional disease, brought on by hard study, over eating and want of exercise; as he was about getting married, he was extremely anxious to get well.— His ailments and the result of the treatment may be learned from his last letter, written sometime after he had ceased to need any further advice from me.

March 19th.

Dear Sir :—I fear that you will think your kind and liberal offer has not been treated with deserved respect by my not writing to you this past winter, the reason was I had nothing particular to communicate.

I have had no soreness or pain in my breast, back, throat or anywhere else this winter, except a slight pain and weakness across my chest when I have had some cold. I have not been troubled with costiveness or piles an hour this winter; I was not free from the former a week last winter, and frequently suffered from the latter. I have had no palpitation since I saw you; I have gained ten or fifteen pounds of flesh; my my strength and activity have in a great measure returned. I have walked eight miles a day, three days in the week without any perceptible fatigue, and sat on my horse from 9 o'clock in the morning until 11 at night, fourteen hours, without the least weariness or thought of being tired. A fair portion of the time I feel as strong as I ever did. My spirits have been better than for several years, and I have less dulness and disposition to sleep in the day time than I ever remember. I have not used a morsel of tobacco since last October, and never expect to use a grain more—the very thought of which gives me comfort. Since my reformation in this respect, I have had no heart-burn, that is an intense burning heat coming up from the stomach, making my throat almost raw, and setting my teeth on edge. I have not suffered much from coldness of hands and feet; your prescriptions have relieved me, if at any time I have been troubled in that respect. My appetite has been uniformly good. I have been out in all sorts of weather, and have cared nothing for storm. I have walked two thirds of a day with my boots full of water, without any ill effect I could perceive on my health. I do not remember being hoarse more than once or twice this winter, and then slightly. I have not missed an appointment, and can speak longer and oftener, with less fatigue, than at any time since I commenced preaching.

If you have leisure to write me a few lines, though nothing special, still your words of encouragement are worth gold to me. I consider that I owe you a debt of gratitude which it is not in my power to discharge. I hope to be in the city soon, when and where I anticipate fulfilling one of your prescriptions not yet attended to, that is to get married."

This gentleman has attended to the last item, and is now an active, efficient minister of the Gospel. When he came to me, he was on the verge of irretrievable ruin of his health, brought on by habits of life impaired by undue exactions of study at Princeton; not the only young man who has come to me direct from a theological seminary, a mere shadow and wreck of what he was when he first entered. I hope the time is not far distant when it shall be considered as essential to have in all our colleges and universities a professor of Hygiene as well as of Morals. Sound morals and sound judgment are inseparable from sound health. No young man ought ever enter the ministry unless he has been well instructed in the general laws of Physiology and Hygiene; from a want of this, four fifths of the educated clergy are, or have been more or less dyspeptic, which never fails to induce an irritability, a waywardness, a changeableness of disposition and temper and a gloom, altogether incompatible with the idea of a perfect minister.

ANOTHER CURE.

The following is an extract from a letter received from a worthy Presbyterian clergyman who had been under my care for some time, and whom I have never seen.

April 11th.

" I have but little cough, my throat is much better. I eat and sleep well enough. Although my time has expired, I hope you will not forsake me. I committed my case into your hands without any knowledge of your personal character, and I have great confidence in your directions. I look upon you, not merely as my physician, but as my friend, &c."

There was, in the main, a great similarity in these last three cases. They were ministers in the same church, with throat affections from like causes, all connected with a dyspeptic condition. The treatment was the same—I directed them

To be out of doors at least five hours daily.

To use a gargle of a saturated solution of alum water, with one sixth tincture of African Cayenne.

To regulate the bowels with one grain each of Turkey Rhubarb and aloes from one to three times a day, with one third of a grain of Sulphate of Iron in each pill or powder.

To use ammoniated liniments to the throat and breast twice a day.

To take once a week a mercurial alterative.

To use cold bread and water only for breakfast and supper ; to eat nothing between meals, and for dinner to use plain, substantial, nourishing food.

In the case before the last, I applied the Nitrate of Silver, sixty grains to the ounce of water, for two weeks daily ; the others I did not see. I enjoined absolute abstinence from tobacco in every form, as useless, indecent, hurtful and destructive, and in the case before the last, the reader will see with what happy results.

492. K. W. G., an Episcopal clergyman, wrote to me complaining of night and morning cough, sore throat, expectoration of heavy yellow matter, repeated attacks of spitting blood within a year past, gasps for breath on excitement, frequent pains betwixt the shoulder blades behind, and had been under treatment some time for consumptive disease; he had had a constant pain in his breast and a settled cough, night sweats, weakness in limbs, great shortness of breath, &c. I prescribed for him nearly a year, with various success, when finally he writes me.

"I am exceedingly gratified at your favorable opinion of my present condition. I truly hope it is as you say; and surely everything tends to confirm the truth of your opinion; if, indeed, I am not already well. I maintain a happy and cheerful frame of mind; a great requisite, as you say. Since my last to you my health has been good; I think better than for the last three years. I still have no cough, although we have lately had a colder spell of weather than any known for years, and I was out in it a great deal of the time, riding and walking. My strength has increased, appetite good, sleep sound, pulse about seventy-six. I have almost constantly some color in my face, not the result of excitement, no flush, and look and feel much like a well man.

I believe I have nothing further to communicate, and as your time is valuable, I will not impose on it. Grateful to you for your kind attentions and the eminent service you have rendered me."

I directed the general treatment in this case; he was using the citrate of iron and a teaspoon of cod liver oil three times a day when he placed himself under my care, and as they did not interfere with my treatment, I allowed him to continue them. What effect they may have had in producing the very favorable termination of the above case I cannot say.

CASES NOT OF CLERGYMEN.

405. W. A. H., New York merchant, writes: age 33, pulse 90. A troublesome cough on getting up in the morning, and sometimes during the day causing nausea and vomiting, has had spitting of blood on several occasions, constipation, very nervous, general chilliness, pains along breast bone and frequent between the shoulder blades; mother died of consumption, has a constant rattling in the throat, had fallen off in flesh. with other minor symptoms. This gentleman got entirely well in a few months, and, as far as I know, remains so to this day. He writes in five weeks after he first applied:

"I am giving the inhaler a trial, and have not lately suffered any inconvenience or pain in my chest, but my cough still hangs on me, and I raise about as usual. Your bitters give me strength and improve my appetite very much. My cough is very troublesome; last evening I coughed a quarter of an hour after retiring, and then fell asleep and did not awake until six this morning. As a general thing, I am improving; though I do not gain strength as fast as I could wish. My friends admire your treatment, and I hope, ere long, to show them of its great virtue. The liniment you sent me is a great deal stronger than what I purchased, it almost takes away my breath when I apply it to my breast. I will continue steadily your advice and shall always read your letters with avidity."

At a later date, in taking leave of me, not having farther use for medical advice, he writes:

"I feel here, in Newburg, in October, as well as I ever did in my life; the ice has frozen a quarter of an inch thick. and the cool, dry atmosphere has braced me up astonishingly. I am quite certain that all disease has disappeared from the chest, and I feel as though the restoration of my health is permanent; certainly, I am quite another being to what I was twelve months ago; my appetite is strong and good, I sleep delightfully, I have more than gained all my flesh. I have not missed your directions since my return from Savannah. I am up here solus, having sent my family to the city.

I must return my unfeigned thanks, that, through your mode of treatment, my health is so fully restored to me; a friend of mine, whom I met recently, and who had not seen me since I began your treatment in May last, remarked to me 'I never saw you better in my life;' of course, this is very flattering to me as well as to yourself."

It has thus been my happiness to restore many to health and to their families in different and distant parts of the country, the pleasure of meeting whom, for the first time, is yet in store for me.

I directed him to use the inhaler, to employ cold water and ammoniacal liniment to the whole surface twice a day, to take a mercurial alterative once in ten days, to go from Savannah, where he had gone for his health, to the high-lands of New York, to use three times a day, an hour before meals, a mixture made thus— thirty grains of sulphate of quinine, and one and a half drams of elixir vitriol in fifteen ounces of rain water.—Dose: one table-spoonful in half-a-glass of water, and nothing more. I gave him nothing for his cough, although he complained of it so often; it gradually disappeared under the general treatment.

NOT CONSUMPTION.

392. A gentleman had a sister to die of consumption, and because he had some cough and pain about the breast, he became alarmed, and came to me for an examination and treatment of his case. I told him his lungs were perfectly sound and that nothing was the matter with him but over eating and want of exercise, and advised him accordingly. In a month he writes:

" I have followed your directions as closely as my circumstances would admit, and I have now the pleasure of informing you that my cough has disappeared and I bèlieve it will not return. I feel as well as I generally feel when I call myself well; I have no pains anywhere, except an occasional one near the left hip bone; my pulse is generally seventy-three, and sometimes less; in fact, if I feel as well as I have done since I saw you, I should have no objection to spending a hundred years here below. The bitterest pill in your prescription is bathing my feet in cold water these frosty mornings, I find it very painful to hold my feet in water below sixty degrees for any length of time; my feelings at present seem to indicate that I shall not need any more medicine.

This case is introduced to show that persons may imagine themselves consumptive and yet be cured perfectly of all their ailments in a few weeks by a simple course of treatment, connected with judicious dieting, which, in a case like the above, is as follows :—

For breakfast and supper, cold bread and butter and cold water; nothing else.

For Dinner:—Take what best agrees with you of plain, nourishing food; one kind of fresh meat broiled or roasted, moderately done, cut up in pieces no larger than a pea before it is put into the mouth, but two kinds of vegetables at one meal, particularly *avoiding* pastries, pies, puddings, cabbage, corn, cucumbers, cakes, dough-nuts, dumplings, fried food of all kinds, hot bread, boiled meats; *using* boiled rice, as on page thirty-eight, sago, tapioca, farina, stale bread, gruels, light soups, boiled turnips, roasted ripe apples and Irish potatoes, tomatoes, eggs soft boiled or whipped, warm corn bread; not a particle of food must be swallowed of any description unless there is a decided desire for it, however weak you may feel, or however long you may have fasted. Nature is the best nurse, and the best judge as to the wants of the system, and the moment the system is prepared to receive nourishment, she will begin to call for it, and will continue to do so until a moderate supply of plain substantial food is taken. Always eat slowly, and never eat anything between meals, on any pretence whatever; before two o'clock in the afternoon, perfect fruits, well ripened, are always admissible and advantageous. Avoid sleeping in the day-time; go to bed at a regular hour, and never remain in bed longer than eight hours at the very farthest, and walk or run two or three miles every day, rain or shine. At dinner-time you may use one glass of cold water, but not a particle of any other liquid whatever. If inclined to be a little costive, drink a glass or two of cold water at once as soon as you get up every morning.

482. Mrs. M. T. came to me in great alarm, fearing that she was falling into con-sumptive disease; complained of weakness and pain in the small of the back, a burning and very severe pain between the shoulder blades behind, oppression in the breast, very great pain at times along the breast bone; a pain in the left side for eighteen months, for which has been blistered, cupped, tartar emetic ointment, and three seatons, and the pain is still there; good deal of general chilliness, a great deal of bad feeling at the pit of the stomach pretty much all the time, feet cold as ice; more or less every day; burning·hands, restless sleep, difficult breathing at times, pal-pitation, night sweats, and spitting blood for a week at a time; ailment came on four years before with chill and bad cough; hoarseness in the throat, and breathing cool air makes it feel raw; the most inconvenient symptoms were pain between the shoulders and in the left side.

With these symptoms I prescribed for this lady, who was married and had several children; and in a few weeks afterwards received the following letter. I have omit-ted to state that she had decided symptoms of stone or gravel.

May 27. —

Dear Sir.—I received your welcome box of remedies in good time. I have not one bad symptom now for every ten when I wrote last. I do not know how to apologise for not writing sooner except by saying I was doing well enough and did not wish to trouble you. I am mending, and you will say fast, when you get through. Why do you think my enormous size would make me unmanageable? You mistake me; I, of course, feel my superiority, but will not be overbearing because of my physical power. It would not do for us all to be small. What would an army of your size do in Mexico? Let city ladies raise the doctors to cure, and we country women the warriors to defend. Were I small, handsome, and accomplished I would be un-fashionable where I live. But, really, I have better hopes of recovery than I have had for four years, and believe if I attend strictly to your directions I will yet be a sound woman, Your book has met the kindest reception wherever it has gone, nearly every neighbor has read it, and think highly of your medical skill, and be assured none are before me in their belief. My husband and children thank you for your attentions. Doctor, I should be glad to hear from you as often as possible. Hoping that you may continue to relieve suffering humanity; I remain, your friend,

MARY T.

At the end of several years this lively correspondent continues to be a healthy woman. When she came to me I told her she had lungs enough for two women, and that none of her symptoms indicated consumptive disease. A strict system of dieting and hepatic remedies, with exercise and cold water bathings, were sufficient.— In cases of this kind, I would rely on the hepatic influence of a pill given every Sunday night, containing from one to two and a half grains of Podophyllin, enough to give two bilious passages in twenty-four hours ; and if in the interval a slight hepatic influence is desirable, give one half a grain daily, or a quarter of a grain three times a day, this is with the exception of *Hydrargiri Chloridum Mite*; the most reliable and safe hepatic remedy known to me ; but it should not be used except under the supervision of a physician who is acquainted with its properties.

NOT ALWAYS SUCCESSFUL.

Lest the reader should begin to imagine that every case that comes under my care gets well, I append the following : I am far from wishing to excite extravagant expectations in any bosom. It will be perceived that scarcely two cases are treated in all respects precisely alike ; the treatment in any case must be according to my judgment, and if that judgment should in any particular case be an erroneous one, I should not only fail to do any good, but might do a great deal of harm ; and feeling conscious that I am as liable to err as other people, I never promise in any case, even the most simple, to do any good whatever ; the utmost that I ever promise, is to do the best I can under the circumstances. I am often appealed to thus, " *Now Doctor I will leave it to you, if you think you can do me any good, I will place myself under your care;*" in all such cases my reply is that I do not think anything about it, and can only say that it is my highest interest to cure you, for if I succeed, others may come through your influence. I will take no such responsibility, nor place it in the power of any one to say *he promised to do so and so and did'nt do it.* Were human nature perfectly honorable and candid, I would act differently; besides, I cannot tell in any case whether my directions would be faithfully observed, nor that the remedies used, unless obtained from me, would be the best of their kind, for it is known to every intelligent and honest Druggist in the Union, that it is next to impossible to obtain a pure article of the most valuable medicines, except in the larger cities, and even there it cannot be done except from a very few established houses. These are evils of such magnitude that Congress has passed a law through the humane influence of one of its members, Doctor Edwards of Ohio, to remedy the outrage; whether it will meet the case, time only can tell. It certainly will prevent adulterated medicines from being brought into this country; but it presents to our own Druggists such increased temptations to the fraud, that it is to be feared that too many will yield to it. For example, Sulphate of Morphine is retailed at common drug stores at the rate of one hundred and twenty dollars a pound, and common flour, which costs but two cents a pound, is mixed with it, and cannot be detected except by a practical chemist or one who has studied the tests. It is very true, that the man who would adulterate an important medicine, is only prevented from stealing by the fear of detection, and such persons have no compunctions in trifling with the lives of the sick and the confiding, when so much money can be made by it, and their detection is almost impossible. It is from these views of the case in part that I am personally the most ultra Homœopathist, and never take medicine, or anything else *as a medicine.* I would rather diet myself a month than swallow a pill or powder or dose of salts or oil, especially as I feel assured that a rigid and literal diet of cold water and cold brown bread would in time cure four fifths of all our diseases, chronic as well as acute. But people do not practically believe this, and are too impatient to submit to such a safe and wholesome mode of cure, but swallow patent medicines by the pound and by the gallon, therefore, and *therefore only*, do physicians live in

E2

palaces, ride in fine carriages, dress in purple and fine linen, and fare sumptuously every day. But to return to the case in hand.

679. vol. 6. R. E. W. writes, Aug. 9th, "I am six feet high and slender, aged 24, pulse 90. Took a chill and fever thirteen months ago ; it became a regular fever and ague in two months, and in six months from the first attack, I had a bad cough, heavy yellow expectoration, night sweats, spitting of blood, sore throat, voice uneven, hoarse and rough, have fallen off forty pounds, am weak, debilitated and emaciated, mother was scrofulous ; I have been salivated, Hydropathized, besides going to an Indian Doctor, great chilliness, cough gives me the most inconvenience, but *I have no pain anywhere.*"

In reply I wrote to him:

" You are in the beginning of consumptive disease. With great diligence and persevering attention to my directions you may recover your health; without that a restoration is impossible. I hope you will spare no pains in doing all I may recommend from time to time, and that you will set about it promptly, for you have no time to lose."

After following my directions about two weeks, he writes :

DEAR SIR:—I do not know that I am any better than I was before I commenced your treatment. I have gained neither strength nor weight ; my cough is very troublesome, especially at night ; the night sweats are not so bad as they were, but still I have some. I had one shake of the ague ; the chills are not so bad as they were. I am also troubled with loose bowels, which has two or three times weakened me down very much. My throat gets sore and hoarse almost every evening, and in the morning it feels well. Your medicine agrees with me very well. I have never felt any uneasiness in my stomach after taking it; I have irregular chills ; in the after part of the night my cough is looser than at any other time, and then I spit up freely ; my appetite is tolerably good, but not as good as it was when I applied to you. I wish you would send me something to strengthen me, I would then have a great deal more satisfaction," &c.

Whether the next letter I receive from this patient will be more favorable, or whether he will become discouraged and stop short off, as some do, is more than I can say. In so serious a disease as an affection of the lungs, that is sometimes for years and years insinuating its poisonous and deadly hold on the system, no one should expect to get well in a week or a month ; or to go on smoothly and regularly to a perfect cure without a hindrance or a draw back ; none should look for recovery except such as can maintain a most resolute determination that if they do die, it will at least not be for the want of trying to get well—such persons generally succeed, when there are comparatively but few chances of recovery, while others not near as bad, die. I hope every one who applies to me will keep this constantly in mind, to wit: the necessity of maintaining all the time a courageous and cheerful resolve that they will get well if possible, in spite of every obstacle.

PRINCIPLES OF TREATING CONSUMPTION.

My whole attention is directed to two points—

To perfect the breathing.

To perfect digestion.

Consumption is always brought on by the impairment of these—it never can be brought on in any other way, and the only mode of cure is to restore these functions to their natural condition.

A man cannot live three weeks without food ; he cannot live three minutes without air. The whole use of food is to make blood, which is every instant carrying renovation and life to every fibre of the human system ; and if for one brief moment the supply were cut off, that fibre would begin to die.

In the process of digestion, all food is divided into two parts, essence and waste ; the latter is regularly carried off, the other is sent to the lungs, where the last process of digestion takes place, by which it is converted into pure blood ; that process is its being exposed to the fresh, pure air that is taken into the lungs at every breath we draw. Without air no new blood can be made, nor can the old blood be renovated. Life, then, consists in a proper amount of the essence of food being exposed to a proper amount of fresh air ; if these proportions are disturbed; disease inevitably invades the system, and health never can be regained, except in the ratio that these proportions are restored.

. To show what an important bearing the breathing and the blood, or rather respiration and circulation, have on our existence, I need only state one fact, that a full grown, healthy man of medium size, must have to flow into his lungs every twenty four hours an amount equal to fifty-seven hogsheads of air, and twenty-four hogsheads of blood.

. And as Consumption always comes on by the respiration and the circulation being hastened, and by this means both are rendered imperfect, the most certain method of detecting the first coming on of Consumption, before it has made any material impression on the system, is to ascertain if the proper quantity of air is received into the lungs at each breath, and just in proportion as the proper quantity is wanting, in such proportion precisely is the unfortunate patient dying; this proportion, as I have already stated, I can determine to the fraction of one cubic inch, and if under my treatment this deficit decreases at every weekly measurement, the patient is daily recovering; but if that deficit increases week after week, death is inevitable in spite of the most favorable symptoms otherwise, and the patient or his nearest friend is at once made acquainted with the fact.

But while so much attention is paid to the condition and function of the lungs, there is one other point equally important, which must never be lost sight of, which is, that the proper amount of the essence of food shall be presented to the air in the lungs, to be made into blood, and that it be of the best material; to do this, the digestive organs must be attended to every day, that they be made to work well; that the food which is presented to them shall be such as will make the most blood in the easiest manner and in the shortest time; and that my patients may always have at hand reliable information as to this important point, I append the following table. which I am not aware has ever been published before, indeed I sent to England for one item in the table, never having seen it in any American book. [See page 80.]

Another most important use to be made of this table is, in reference to the condition of the bowels; the rule is this, when the bowels are loose, such things should be eaten as have the least waste matter to be carried off over the surface of the tender and inflamed bowels; such food, with absolute rest, that is, lying down on a bed or sofa twenty-three hours out of every twenty-four, will cure very many cases of loose bowels, while food that has a great deal of waste, would hurry on to a fatal issue in a few hours; the reader can note the difference—Rice properly boiled, has eighty-eight parts of nutriment and twelve of waste, while cucumbers have two parts of nutriment, and ninety-eight of waste; the most common nurse will tell you that *rice is binding*, although ignorant of the cause of it, that it is nearly all nutriment, and has almost no waste; hence the universal rule of diet in times of cholera, should be to eat such things as have the least waste, which, with regular rest, avoiding mental and bodily excitement, remaining quietly within doors a great part of the time, never exercising to weariness, these I fully believe, are a perfect exemption from cholera in its worst epidemic ragings. I was in New Orleans in December, 1848, when it began its ravages there, and remained there until May ensuing, when I went direct to Cincinnati, and remained there during the whole time of its presence, and I am not sensible that during all that weary period, from December 18th, 1848 to August of '49, that I ever had the most remote symptom of a cholera affection, beyond what quietude would remove, and the principles of diet above named would keep away; and among all my patients, who for themselves and families would naturally ask my advice as to the best course of conduct to be pursued, not one single death from cholera, not even a single case of cholera has occurred, as far as I know or believe, and that too, though scattered a thousand miles asunder; in addition, my standing advice has been, not to take an atom of the simplest medicine if attacked, but to send for a physician in whom confidence could be reposed; but if there was no prospect of getting one in two hours, and there was vomiting or cramps, or any kind of discharge from the bowels oftener than once in two or three hours, I counselled them to take twenty grains of calomel in two pills of ten grains each, and wait quietly until the physician came, this will remain on the stomach when nothing else will, and usually, within two hours, *stops all passages*, and in ten hours from the time taken, dark or green passages appear, and the patient is safe, if let alone; to eat as much ice as he chooses, and as much boiled rice as there is an appetite for, and not an atom more. No one thing, no one course will always cure in cholera, as every sensible man must know ; no one remedy is in all cases applicable or possible; but the treatment I have named is, I think, as often effectual as any other one plan. I have thus digressed purposely for the benefit of such as may have this publication, in case the dreadful scourge may visit us again. Taking things to prevent cholera, leaving home during its prevalence, either for business or safety, or making great or sudden changes in one's usual mode of life, are all in my opinion equally injudicious and fatal in their tendencies and operations. Every step a man takes, every half mile, he rides on horse or in carriage or steamboat, tends in my opinion to bring on cholera in cholera times. While the epidemic is present in a community, I would advise every one whose ordinary habit is to have one action from the bowels every twenty-four hours, to consider himself as having cholera, if he has less than one passage in twenty-four hours, or if he have more than two passages in twenty-four hours ; in either case, go home, lie down, eat nothing, drink nothing, take nothing, but send at once for a physician who has your confidence, and wait until he comes. Remember that in cholera times, unusual constipation is as certainly cholera as unusual looseness ; I believe those cases are the most speedily fatal where the looseness is preceded by constipation for one, two or more days, consequently instead of feeling a greater degree of safety when you are costive, at such times you should feel greater alarm than if you had moderate and gradual looseness of bowels. These opinions may appear novel to many, and even to some medical men; but I think close observation will convince them of their truthfulness.

OBSERVATIONS ON THROAT DISEASE.

In the large majority of persons in this country there is a *Tubercular Diathesis,* that is, a tendency to consumptive disease; and whenever, in any particular man, there is such a tendency, that disease will fall upon that part of the body most weakened, whatever may be the cause of its being weakened; just as in a common mill-dam, wherever there is the slightest break there the whole force of the current tends. If, then, a man has a consumptive or tubercular tendency, and his lungs are weakened by a very bad cold, or by impure air, or by any other means, the whole force of the tubercular current drives to that point, and he falls a victim to consumption of the lungs; if the bowels be the weak part, tubercles form there, and he has chronic diarrhœa and finally death; if the mesenteric glands are weakened, they become tuberculated, harden, prevent the nutriment passing into the system, and there is negro consumption, a general wasting away, a drying up of all the powers of life, and the man dies like the burning out of a candle; and if the upper part of the windpipe, the voice making organs are irritated or weakened by any means whatever; tubercles form there, becking, hemming, hawking, frequent clearing, or swallowing, or pricking, or dryness, or rawness, or burning, or itching, or tickling come on, then hoarseness, ulceration, and death.

In very many instances this throat disease comes on, not by a destruction of the parts, but simple irritation of the mucous membrane ; if let alone, and the causes are kept up, other changes as inevitably follow, as that the shadow follows the sun, congestion, inflammation, swelling, destruction.

In cases of this kind the cause must be discovered, then removed, and next, such other things done as will be best calculated to change the diseased condition and remove it.

My practice, then, in cases of throat disease, consists mainly in three things.

1. To discover the cause of the throat ail, and to remove it.

2. To bring all the secretories of the system up to the healthful standard, and keep them there.

3. To make such appliances to the parts as may be judged best adapted in each particular case, to break down the present diseased action, and harden them against future attacks.

As to the first ; if the cause of the disease is discovered *in its beginnings,* the throat will get well of itself.

As to the second ; when more advanced, general constitutional means are all that is necessary.

As to the third; I have only to say, that I rely mainly upon the gargles recommended by Allopathic or old-school standard writers.

I never have used as a gargle, nor do I think anything could justify its use, any preparation, however weak, of the nitrate of silver, because it is utter destruction to the teeth, and there are many things very much better.

NITRATE OF SILVER,

Applied by means of a sponge or otherwise, is used by many. I have sometimes used it to advantage, but I no not consider it a very valuable remedy, and do not often use it, because :—

1. Persons have come to me to be cured, after having had it applied, to no purpose, for weeks and months.

2. I consider it utterly impossible for a person to apply it to the voice making organs in his own case.

3. Nitrate of silver, alone, is not sufficient to cure any case.

4 By persons relying upon it alone, valuable time is often lost, the disease progresses to the lungs, and all is over.

5. I believe it is at this time the means of destroying human life, and will continue so to do, until there is a more general and correct understanding as to the nature, character, and symptoms of diseases of the throat and lungs.

The way human life is daily sacrificed by the use of nitrate of silver, is as follows: Many, very many persons have a cough, that cough is immediately excited by a tickling or other sensation in the throat, oftenest, perhaps, at the little hollow at the bottom of the neck in front, and having no unusual sensation lower down, they conclude that it cannot be any other than a throat affection, and begin to apply the nitrate; forgetting, that sometimes the point of feeling is far distant from that where the actual mischief lies, as in striking the elbow the unpleasant sensation is felt at the finger ends; in the same way, a tickling in the throat is very often caused by diseased action going on deep down in the lungs.

My own opinion as to the worth of the nitrate of silver in diseases of the throat is simply this, that in the hands of a discriminating and skilful physician, it is in some cases a *valuable aid* in the treatment of such affections, and no more; and I think that sober, old practitioners all over the country will bear me out in this assertion.

Clergyman's sore throat is a phrase calculated to mislead, because in my own experience, a larger number of persons, in proportion, in the common walks of life have throat ail than of clergymen; the truth is, as far as my own observation extends, throat affections more frequently arise from a dyspeptic condition, than from any other cause; hence my success in the treatment of so many cases of so called *Bronchitis*, in persons whom I have never seen, or have seen but once. In none of these cases can the nitrate do any permanent good, unless the disordered digestion be rectified; when that is done, the throat gets well of itself without the argentine solution.

But, after all, these throat ails do but too frequently end in Consumption and death; see page 18, simply because they are neglected at first; people feel that it is almost bordering on the ridiculous, to be placing themselves in the hands of a physician for so slight an ailment, when they can eat, and sleep, and walk about the streets, and, to all appearance, look as healthy as other men.

When there is a consumptive tendency, and the general health is feeble, although there be no cough, no pain in the breast, the slightest unnatural sensation about the throat, continuing for a month or more, should excite the liveliest alarm.

When these diseases are in a family connexion, the members of the family, whose modes of life are similar, are attacked successively as they approach the same age, and are safe in proportion as that age is past.

When any member of a family has had either of these diseases, the slightest symptoms of them in any other member of the family should be regarded with apprehension, and prompt attention should be given to their removal and eradication; this is so easily done, if attempted at first, and so generally admitted, too, that such frequent and gross neglect and, procrastination cannot be accounted for except in one way, people have such a horror of undertaking a *course of medicine*, as they term it: yet most inconsistently they will turn right round and take the advice of any old granny they meet with, or any body else, provided it be not a respectable physician; and buy and swallow, for weeks and months, whole dozens of bottles of drops, syrups, balsams, and the like; they will go through a course of medicine, and some of them through a dozen courses, if, as at meals, each kind is a course, on their own responsibility, and yet dread a course under the superintendence of a physician. I do not complain of this, but merely state it as a reason why slight throat ailments end so often in death; persons either neglect them because they seem so trivial, or lose time while they are experimenting with their health and lives by the advice of ignorant people, or from a horror of *going through a course of medicine*; but in the early stages of which I am speaking a course of medicine is the very thing which they least need, and which is most likely to infix the disease.

In very many cases, however, the lungs themselves have been diseased before hand, and the throat becomes affected in the progress of the disease; sometimes the disease appears in both places at once, and finally fixes itself in the weaker part; but mark it well, that most generally whether the disease is deepest in the throat or lungs, the throat, having most sensibility, complains the most, if not wholly, the inconvenience there is so great as to distract the attention from the lungs altogether, the patient feels, in comparison, almost nothing there, because the distress in the throat is so great, while, if that were entirely removed, the lung affection would at once excite alarm; thus, too, it happens that sometimes the throat appears to be the whole cause of death, when on examination, after death, the lungs prove to have extensively decayed away; but it is impossible to make such a mistake by the mode of examination which I have adopted; if the lungs are at all impaired, even to a slight extent, it can not escape detection.

Sometimes the upper parts of the throat are affected like the other end of the alimentary canal in the disease called piles, the blood-vessels of the rectum become inflamed, congested, and burst, blood is discharged, and there is a perfect relief for days, weeks, and months; there are cases in which the blood-vessels in the regions about the back part of the throat and top of the windpipe and gullet become periodically or irregularly turgid, at last break, blood flows out, and relief follows without ill consequences.

Sometimes there is an ailment in throat from some difficulty along the tract of the alimentary canal. The stomach is out of order, or there is constipation, and the throat complains although so far distant; at other times, the other end, the rectum, complains from the very same cause, giving piles to one man and intolerable itching to another, especially after getting into the bed at night; why a stomach affection should make itself felt at the extreme ends in different persons it is not so important to know as that it is a fact.

At other times the throat ail is a purely nervous affection and can only be cured by constitutional remedies adapted to particular cases.

So close is the connection between throat ail and Consumption, that sometimes the hoarseness and sore throat precede Consumption and sometimes they follow it; it is, therefore, a matter of the very highest importance in all throat affections of several weeks standing, to determine definitely whether the lungs are sound and whole, working healthfully and freely, and I am fully convinced in my own mind that this cannot be done with any approach to certainty, except in the manner practised by me; to wit: by ascertaining to a single inch the mathematical measurement of the lungs.

In some instances a man feels and appears perfectly well in every respect, has no pain, no irregularity in any of the bodily functions, if you look into the throat there is no appearance of any kind of inflammation, nor can it be told from the pulse that anything is the matter; but something very serious is the matter and this is apparent to the most careless observer when the man speaks, for he is hoarse, or speaks with difficulty, and in some instances cannot possibly speak above a whisper; there is simple *Aphonia* or *voicelessness*. This is a serious ailment, because it is very difficult to cure; seatons, issues, nauseants, leeches, sores made by croton oil, or tartar emetic plasters, low diet, none of these things do any good. This form of disease depends on the atonic condition of the voice making organs, and perhaps, in part, a weakened condition of the laryngial muscles. In such cases nitrate of silver does no more good, and not so much as cold water, if freely gargled with; the cure consists in applying constitutional means previously refered to.

CURIOUS FACTS ABOUT DIGESTION.

Some very singular items have been noticed in reference to digestion, and it may be as serviceable as singular to record some of them here, as they are of great practical utility.

Red meats, such as beef, lamb, mutton &c., are more easily digested and are more nutritious than the white meats, such as chicken, fish, and the like, and yet a broiled chicken is good for an invalid or weak stomach, when a piece of roast beef, or beef steak would be productive of serious consequences, simply because red meats are more stimulating, excite the pulse, and increase or bring on fever, while chicken and other white and young meats have a far less stimulating effect.

Oils and fat meats are the most nutritious of all articles of food, more so than soft boiled rice, or brown bread, and require three or four hours for digestion, and yet a piece of fat meat, which a child dying of summer complaint will eat ravenously, will sometimes cure the child and fatten it up wonderfully.

Fat bacon, fat midlings fried and eaten for breakfast, a very common dish in all the west, is an excellent remedy for a person, who in common language is said to be "bilious."

Many cases of torpid liver and indigestion are cured by fat meats and oils, by the same means persons who complain of being *weakly*, of *falling away*, of loosing their flesh, sometimes get fat.

I do not know certainly what is the reason of all this, but inasmuch as it is known, that when oily food is used the bile assists in its digestion, it may be that there is something in the nature of oil to excite the liver into action, or to draw the bile into the stomach. I have certainly by administering fatty matters led persons to gain in strength, and increase in flesh three, five, seven pounds in a week, to get a good appetite and regular bowels, when before they complained of weakness, no appetite, sick stomach, and constipated bowels. These are facts, the theory must take care of itself.

For the same reason persons convalescing, or after being purged are allowed simple soups and not meat, while the latter is more easily digested, but the soups containing more oil promote perhaps the gentle flow of bile.

The gastric juice is essential to digestion, it is caused to flow into the stomach as soon as any substance is introduced into the stomach, whether it be a piece of leather or a pieee of beef steak ; this juice contains an acid, and the more indigestible any article of food is, the greater amount of sourness does the gastric juice contain, hence when persons eat something that *does not agree* with them, that is, not easily digested, they say *it soured on the stomach*, or complain of *heart burn*. The use to make of this is, whatever article of food is followed by *sour stomach* or *heart burn*, that article is hard of digestion to that stomach and ought to be avoided altogether, at least it should be taken in diminished quantity. But do not forget that different stomachs *bear* different things ; and what disagrees with you to day, may agree very well next week or next month, and the stomach *must be humored* however fickle it may seem.

Sometimes however, shall I not say nearly always, people eat so much that there is not gastric juice, or acid enough to digest the food, then it ferments, produces belching, colicky pains, sick stomach and the like, therefore, common vinegar, which has more of the properties of the gastric juice than any other known substance is often used to very great advantage, especially by persons who have weak stomachs, to aid the stomach in digesting articles which are known to be difficult of digestion hence vinegar is plentifully used with cabbages, raw or boiled, with cucumbers &c., hence too is it that catsups of various kinds are eaten, and sour krout almost digested by the vinegar it contains, before it is eaten. Hence too it is, that some cases of loose bowels are cured by eating plentifully of good ripe tart fruits uncooked, as they supply sourness to digest these undigested articles of food which give rise to the diarrhœas that are not of a billious character. Hence too, a good ripe apple or two, a little sour, after a hearty breakfast or dinner is advantageous rather than otherwise, provided not much more than the juice is swallowed, the better plan by far however is not to eat so much as to require an apple to save us from the effects of our imprudence.

The connection between the various symptoms of consumptive disease and the influence which one diseased condition has in effecting another is wonderful. There are really three processes of digestion, the first occurs in the stomach, the second along the tract of the intestines, and the third and last in the lungs; this process is carried on by incessant motion of the three parts named, and when either of these cease their motions permanently we die. If the lungs cease to act altogether, we perish in three minutes; if the bowels in common language become "torpid," we take on sickness, fever and death in a few days unless they are aroused by some means or other. In health the bowels are as incessant in their workings as the waves of the ocean, during every instant of our whole existence, and the instant they cease we begin to die; if for example a bullet penetrates the abdomen and pierces a bowel it becomes quiescent that moment and death is inevitable within four or five days, generally within two, a bullet may pass through the lungs, or be lodged in the heart and the man may get well and live many years; but he never survives a bullet penetration of the bowels, because that instant they cease to move; a state of activity then is a state of health as far as the bowels are concerned, they are kept in motion by three means which I shall name.

By the stimulus of the food passing through them.

By the motion of our bodies, exercise for example of any kind.

By the motion of the lungs in breathing, for in every breath we draw, an undulating movement is imparted thereby to the whole of the intestines. But there are times when a man is liable to be without food for hours and days and weeks, for he can live twenty days without food in rare instances; then the bowels not having their natural stimulus would stagnate and we would die if there were no other means to keep them in motion.

As to the second means, we do not exercise in our sleep and the very first night the seeds of death would be sown in us if the bowels were wholly dependent on bodily exercise for their activity.

But if we are starving for weeks, and if in addition we are confined for months by lingering disease, or bound to a prison floor by chains for years together, yet we always breathe every instant of our existence, as ceaselessly as that Kind Eye that never sleeps in its vigil for the happiness of His earth born children.

But when the lungs begin not to breathe free enough, the bowels do not receive their proper motion, digestion becomes deficient, the blood poor, the strength fails, the body wastes away and the man dies.

It is the whole end and aim in my system of treatment to detect this deficient lung working in its very incipiency and to lend all my energies to bring them back to their natural healthful action—in proportion as I succeed in doing this, men get well, and as certainly as this is not done they die.

RESPIRATION—CIRCULATION.

Consumption progresses with an equal pace with the increased acceleration of the pulse and the breathing, and their connection is indissoluble.

All consumptive persons are chilly; they cannot bear cold; the cold "strikes through" them; when they go out of doors, if the weather is at all cold, the cold chills run over them, especially are they felt along the back bone; this is the case even while they have a feverish pulse, and the skin feels hot and dry. Why is this? It is because the body and blood are kept warm by the oxygen contained in the air we breathe, uniting with the carbon in the blood returned to the right side of the heart and the essence of the food which is mixed with the returned blood, they both entering the right side of the heart together. Now, however much a person may eat, he is nourished, strengthened and warmed only in proportion as there is a due supply of oxygen, and as this can only be brought in by means of the air breathed into the lungs, it is plain that if the lungs are half gone or inoperative, there will be only half enough heat, and so in any other proportion down to one two hundredth part. The reader must perceive then how extremely interesting it must be to be able to detect these derangements in their far off comings; and furthermore to be able to measure their disappearance under appropriate treatment with mathematical precision. It is wonderful to me that these things are regarded with so much indifference. I did think that the mere statement of them would have speedily aroused the most eager and intense inquiry. I abhor hobbies, and therefore do not feel authorized to go farther than to make these simple announcements. A man need only think, and he will at once be enchained to the subject.

I said that if the lungs are partly gone, they cannot resent enough oxygen to the' blood to generate a sufficient heat for the system, if then the lungs cannot take in air enough, it is a matter of the utmost advantage that the air inspired should contain the largest possible amount of oxygen, to do this, it should, in the first place, be as pure as possible, in the next place, it should be condensed, for the more condensed it is, the more oxygen there is in each cubic inch of bulk; but the way to condense air is to make it cold, hence cold air is best for consumptives, provided it is dry, for it warms and purifies the blood in proportion as it is cold and dry— that is condensed and pure—but in the south where consumptives gather from all parts of the Union by a kind of universal advice and consent, the climate being warm, the air is rarified, and in addition is filled with various miasms, and still more, a very large portion of the time the weather is damp rainy, or foggy, and the air is loaded with vapors before it goes into the lungs, and consequently cannot absorb the moisture already there waiting to be conveyed away by each supply of breath; consequently there is an accumulation of moisture in the lungs, and there is dullness and oppression, that in some instances, makes life a burden to the invalid, for hours become years. The necessity for dry air to be taken into the lungs to absorb the moisture waiting there for it, will be felt when it is remembered that a person of ordinary size does in each twenty-four hours, throw off from the lungs by expiration nearly one pint and a quarter of water, and it is easy to conceive how greatly a person must feel oppressed, if but a small part of a pint and a quarter of water is in the lungs beyond what is natural.

Damp weather, then, not only oppresses the system, diminishing the liveliness of the circulation ; it not only, as above stated, prevents the generation of heat enough to keep off chilliness, but this very dampness, in addition, carries off from the surface a larger amount of the insufficient quantity of heat already generated, than dry air would do ; if you dip your hand in water, hot or cold, in summer or winter, and hold it up, it will feel cooler than the other hand kept dry, showing that moisture conducts away the heat from the system more rapidly than dryness, therefore consumptive people who always feel too chilly, or at least are too easily chilled, should not live in a damp, foggy or rainy climate, nor be exposed to damp winds; all these things abound in the south in the winter, and yet consumptives flock there from every point of the compass to get well, but in reality to die the sooner.

But there is another practical ill effect to a consumptive living in a damp climate, or where he is exposed to cold raw winds, such as always follow rains in the south in the winter time, and such as are constantly felt on the borders of all prairies, lakes or sea shores after rains. The gastric juice dissolves food and digests it quicker and more perfectly when it is of a higher temperature, than when it is of a lower ; but it is known by actual experiment and observation, as detailed by Dr. Beaumont, that when the day is damp, the temperature of the inside of the stomach was as low as ninety-four degrees by Farenheit's Thermometer, but when the weather was clear, dry and cool, it rose to one hundred degrees, and on exercise, to one hundred and three.

I have always contended that consumptive persons should live in a cool, dry atmosphere, not in a warm, damp one—and that they will live longer by a free exposure to the dry cold of midwinter every day, and I even say rain or shine, than if they are confined to rooms that are regulated to a degree. It is the cool air that brings life back again, because it is pure, condensed and nutritious, and it is the warm air that hurries the invalid to the grave, because it is rarified and full of malaria, damps and miasms.

A TRUTHFUL DESCRIPTION.

The following extracts of letters, written to me by persons who had read my book, will show that the descriptions which I have given of the symptoms of throat and lung affections are truthful, natural, and convincing; they show farther that my book has also answered the objects designed by me wherever it has been read, viz:—

It has drawn attention to existing symptoms in their infancy.

F

It has enabled persons to discover the character of the disease with which they were threatened.

It has led them to apply to me promptly.

LETTER ONE.   Chillicothe, May 25.

A friend of mine has lately met with a work of yours on diseases of the throat and lungs, and from some cases you have described, she is led to believe that her throat is more diseased than her liver or lungs. She would like to know your opinion without delay.

LETTER TWO.   Armstrong Co., Pa., June 1.

Having accidentally obtained a copy of your publication, 1 have therein found described, under the head of *Laryngitis*, a disease which has afflicted my wife for the last two and one-half years. She has consulted several physicians and none of them appeared to understand the disease, or describe the symptoms as accurately as your publication; your description of *Laryngitis* coincides in every particular with her disease, unless it is that her tongue has partially lost its power, becomes apparently exhausted in talking; also a soreness between the shoulders, or more under the left one, which frequently becomes painful. By your description she thinks her disease has not arrived at an advanced state, but it still continues to become worse; it apparently ceases, then renews its attacks every few days. She has yet no cough; her stomach has been dyspeptic for the last eight or ten years. Please give directions, &c.

LETTER THREE.   Knox Co., Indiana, June 22.

I have examined your publication, and desire to know your terms, &c. There are also two young men of my acquaintance to whom I showed your book, and they have desired me to write to you. They have been taking medicines from physicians and syrups of different kinds for the last five years, without any benefit; they are still taking sarsaparilla syrup; they are yet attending to their business, but are not capable of performing much labor.

I was attacked myself, some twenty months ago, with a severe cough and some of the symptoms of Consumption; it left me in three or four months and I experienced no more inconvenience from it, until last March, when I had occasional attacks of sore throat, without any appearance of taking a cold or having a cough, but a constant disposition to clear the throat of a tough-like substance, more particularly when first going to bed at night or getting up in the morning, with a tickling in the throat, no symptom of yellow matter perceivable; the same symptoms still continue.

LETTER FOUR.   Meigs, O., June 26.

Your publication came into my hands a few weeks ago; my wife, from the information detailed in your book, thinks that she has *Bronchitis*. As she cannot visit you at present, and as persons may be cured without visiting your office, please write, &c.

LETTER FIVE.   Corydon, July 5.

I have examined your book, in which are so plainly described the various diseases of the throat and lungs, that I am led to think you could do me good if you had a correct description of the manner in which I am diseased. You say that a blank form is sent to persons who cannot visit you, by means of which the disease may be thoroughly described. I think it is what you call *Laryngitis*. I have a cough and spit up heavy in the mornings, voice failing. Please send me the form.

Your strong friend, &c.

LETTER SIX.   College Corner, Aug. 2.

By accident your pamphlet came into my hands, and after giving it a perusal, I am anxious that you should prescribe for myself and companion, She is predisposed to Consumption, inheriting it from her father, who died with it while young, but she has none of the symptoms as yet, with the exception of shortness of breath on any little over exercise, and a slight cough which has bothered her for several months back, but it is unattended with any pain and she seldom raises any kind of matter. She has taken medicine from two physicians, but they only prescribed something to allay the cough, stating that she had not Consumption.

With regard to myself, I have what I think is *Laryngitis*, brought on by indigestion, a slight affection of the liver, and a falling of the palate, which came down about four years ago, and caused a slight tickling in my throat and hawking. I had a piece of my palate taken off a short time ago; the dry tickling has ceased, but there is still a collection of white matter which causes hecking. There is a sore place on the right side of Adam's apple.

RECAPITULATION.

CAUSES OF THE THROAT DISEASE.

Frequently renewed colds, sharp cry, forced exercise of the voice, blows, falls, wounds, chills, foreign bodies, sudden suppression of any breakings out on the skin, habitual exercise of the voice in public speaking, teaching and singing, immoderate venery, masturbation, syphilis, cancer, tumors, wet feet, sleeping in a draft of air, sitting on cold or damp seats, suppression of periodical turns, stretching of the neck, such as plastering or painter's graining require.

SYMPTOMS.—Frequent clearing of the throat; disposition to swallow, as if to clear away something, but as soon as the swallowing is over, the sensation returns; hoarseness; cracked voice; inability to speak above a whisper; slight pricking sensation in swallowing, sometimes pain; inability to swallow liquids, and sometimes solids; scalding sensation in the throat; feeling of pain running up the side of the neck, sometimes extending to the ear, giving more or less of an ear-ache; a heavy or hurting kind of feeling at the bottom of the neck; a feeling of tenderness about the top of the windpipe, under the jaws and forward; sensation of great dryness, or heat in the back part of the throat; a scraping sensation about the swallow; a slight hacking cough; in the last stages of the disease, mouthfuls of yellow matter are brought up easily without coughing; pain on pressing the side or front of the throat or in turning the head much or suddenly.

No one case has half of these symptoms, most cases have three or four or more; some have only one symptom. Any one symptom, continuing "off and on" for weeks, should be regarded with serious alarm, this disease being only second in insidiousness, intractability and fatality, to Consumption itself, unless treated properly in its first beginnings.

THE PRINCIPLES ADVOCATED.—Consumption admits of cure in its last stages, but this is of such rare occurrence that it ought never to be promised, and is seldom to be hoped for.

When the lungs have begun to decay, a cure is doubtful, unless the person have a strong constitution, or the decay is small.

In the first stages of Consumption, before the lungs have begun to decay, or before tubercles have become numerous, the disease admits of an easy, and perfect and permanent removal in a large majority of cases, with but little internal medicine, no confinement to the house; and without the use of blisters or running sores.

No person can be certainly pronounced to have Consumption, (until it has advanced to its hopeless stages,) without the use of the new diagnostic to which I have made reference in these pages.

I possess the means of indicating, with certainty, the first approaches of consumptive disease, and hence the cure also, at this stage.

I measure the power and extent of the lungs with mathematical precision.

No person can take on Consumption without a previous loss of lung power.

When the lungs have lost their capability of regaining their lost power, and that power is still diminishing, the patient must inevitably die, however well and strong he may feel in every respect.

The loss, the diminution, the gain, are indicated in a manner which does not admit of mistake, in conjunction with the general principles of auscultation.

When persons under my care are increasing their lung force, I encourage them to remain, because I believe they are getting well; when in the course of two or three weeks there is no increase, under the use of appropriate means, and no diminution in the rapidity of respiration and arterial action, I dismiss them, because I believe they must die, and they ought to be at home.

I never knew a person to die of Consumption, within a year, who possessed his appropriate lung power, (as determined by me,) at the time of his examination, except in one instance, 497, and this was under extraordinary circumstances.

No person in my care has ever recovered when, within a month, he has failed, under appropriate means, to regain a portion of his lost lung power, or to diminish arterial action and respiration.

Persons who have lost one third of their lung power, have got well, by regaining the whole of it, while under my care, and are well to this day.

If the capability of regaining lost lung power is lost, and respiration and arterial action cannot be reduced to something near the natural standard, the patient must inevitably die of Consumption ; this point is usually determined within a month.

When this capability is lost, no amount of effort will regain a particle ; when it is not lost, easy efforts make a gain, which is usually perceptible within a fortnight.

In mere throat disease, there is no loss in lung power ; when the lungs are affected, even slightly, there always is a loss of lung power.

I believe this new diagnostic, in connection with rational auscultation, will always give a correct answer to the question, in any case : " Does Consumption exist in any stage or not."

I have learned to be sanguine in nothing ; to be surprised at nothing ; to be willing to consider anything that properly comes within my sphere ; I have seen the folly of becoming absorbed in one idea, and running away with it ; but in reference to this new method of determining the existence of Consumption, the mode of treating this disease, and of curing throat ail, I may safely say, that they open up a new field of enquiry, that many a valuable life will be saved thereby, and that every year, physicians and others will look upon them with diminished prejudice and increasing favor.

When I have had a longer time for making observations, of adding to their variety, and of of contemplating the permanency of results, I purpose throwing it before the community in full, and trust thereby, that I will be able to do some good to the world I live in.

I wish to direct very special attention to some remarks about to be made in reference to Consumption ; many have been hastily abandoned, and have died in consequence of their neglect, who otherwise might have lived.

A person never dies from a first or single attack of Consumption. Persons generally get well of one, two, three, or more attacks of this disease ; but each attack weakens and impairs the constitution, and these continuing to follow one another, there is at length a wreck and ruin of the whole. I mean by an attack of Consumption, as follows :

From causes previously named, tubercles, which may be termed the seeds of Consumption, form about the lungs ; not over the lungs generally, but in small patches or clusters, as large as a half dime piece, and many times larger ; between these patches the lungs are healthy and sound ; these patches of tubercles would produce no inconvenience, if they did not ripen ; that is, enlarge, turn yellow, and run together a liquid mass, as small shot if laid side by side on a shovel on the fire, will run together. When this ripening process commences, by the tubercles beginning to increase in size, preparatory to softening, the person begins to cough more, and he thinks he has taken a fresh cold ; as the mass becomes more liquid, it moves more or less by change of position, or by the air, in breathing, passing through it ; this motion causes it to act, as any other foreign body would act in the lungs, a crum of bread for example ; that is, produces a tickling sensation, which causes irrepressible cough ; this cough is an effort of nature to rid the lungs of this foreign, irritating, inflaming substance ; it is an effort of nature to cure the patient ; as soon as it is all out, the cough subsides, and the patient begins to get well ; just as a bile begins to get well when all the matter is removed from it, *and never before.* Tubercles ripen in spots, as berries do in a berry patch. But, unfortunately, no sooner is the patient rid of one ripening process, feels better, and begins to hope anew, when another cluster begins to ripen, and the same process has to be gone over again ; and thus it is in ceaseless successsion for months, and even years sometimes, until the poor suffering body is wearied and worn to a skeleton, and death at last ends the tedious conflict.

This is the case where there are a number of patches of tubercles, in different parts of the lungs. But sometimes, from causes unknown to us, there is but a single patch, while the lungs in every other part are perfectly sound. In a case like this, a person goes through all the symptoms of regular Consumption, more or less violent, according to the size of the patch, and strength of his constitution; and when the last remnant of matter is coughed up, the cough ceases, the system gets repose, gains strength, and the man gets permanently well, because there is no other patch of tubercles to carry him through similar process. The most of constitutions are able to go through several such attacks; any one, on reflection, will find that those whom he has known to die of Consumption, did not do so until they had gotten better and worse many times, and the appearance of the lungs after death confirms this view of the case.

My practice, then, is to sustain the constitution, to watch over it, and give it all the strength possible, while it is passing through these attacks, in the hope, that each one may be the last; hence, there ought to be perseverance against every obstacle, *until death!* unless the lungs are more than half gone, with no constitution to go upon; or, unless they were very extensively covered with tubercles over the upper half, on both sides of the breast; in either case there is no rational ground for hope. Under this view of the case, it has already occurred to the reflecting reader, what an utterly mischievious practice it is to take medicines to subdue the cough. It is the presence of the yellow matter which nature seeks to get rid of by the cough; for there can be no healing process going on as long as it is there; on the contrary, it sets up irritation, inflammation, fever, hectic, night sweats, loose bowels, and all the other most wasting elements of the hateful disease. Every druggist knows that there is no patent cough remedy which does not have opium in it, in some shape or other. It lulls for awhile, and the person thinks himself better, because the cough abates; but the yellow matter of softened tubercles is still rankling in his vitals, and gaining additional power of ill, until the dose has to be increased or repeated oftener, and such are the directions on all the cough medicines I ever saw, "*gradually increase the dose!*" until finally not less than a large part of a bottle, at once, does any good at all; or the stomach becomes so "set against it," that the patient turns away from it in disgust. Hence it is, that persons have come to me, saying, in reference to some particular remedy, "I have taken whole tub-fulls of it."

It is under this view of the case, that I have so often said in these pages, that I give little or no medicine for Consumption itself; no medicine can reach the lungs, to have any healing effect on them; as I think no medicine can do the lungs any real good, except so far as it has a tendency to render regular and healthful the various functions of the human body, and thus, in the only safe and natural way giving, not a fictitious and transitory, but a natural and lasting strength to the body, enabling it to sustain itself against the attack of tubercular softenings just spoken of; and every respectable physician, every scientific druggist, knows it as well as he does his a, b, c's, that opium in any shape, and in any quantity, has, in all its tendencies, a deranging effect on every natural function of the human machine; and that when it does afford strength, it is only for a moment, and then lets the system proportionably lower down.

Medical men may rest assured, that the great engine in the treatment of Consumption, is to sustain the system in each debilitating attack; not by any secret remedy, not by any specific, or magic-working compound, but by *the general principles of established practice*, to accomplish an object by means, by expedients, by substitutes, as varying as the varying constitutions and predominant ailments of each particular case. Sustain the system on *general principles*, and nature will cure the Consumption herself, by her own inherent powers, with the aid of external appliances and physical means, if there is constitution enough to go upon, without bandages and braces, and supporters, and other devices, which ignorant and designing men are daily preparing, to make money out of, making their instruments, and then forming a theory, out of pure imagination, to fit them. Having thus stated my views, any intelligent man, especially a physician, must see how impossible it is to frame any mode of treatment, for the cure of Consumption, adapted even to a majority of cases, in a manner to allow persons to practice on themselves, and they must further see, how utterly absurd it is to suppose, that any one medicine or remedy could be named, which could possibly be used as a general rule, *in common hands.* No intelligent medical man, can possibly take up a book, however much it promises, with the expectation of finding in it any one remedy, for the general cure of Consumption- It

is a disease in which the whole constitution is involved; in which every bodily function is more or less deranged; and to treat it successfully, the whole system of medical
practice must be most thoroughly understood; not the understanding which theories
and books give, but the understanding acquired by long years of close, correct and extended observation, of actual occurrences at the bed-side, together with another indis-
pensible requisite, the exercise of a sound judgment. These alone are worth all the
books, and theories, and medical schools in the universe; for these can make a safe
and successful practitioner, and these only.

That Consumption in its last stage, that is, when the lungs themselves are actually
decaying, admits of arrest and cure, and that the patient may die many years after,
of some other disease, is considered in these pages as an established fact, a demonstrable truth; and I know of no modern medical writer on lung affections, of eminence and respectability, who thinks otherwise. The people generally do not believe
that Consumption can be cured, and many physicians are of the same opinion; but
the views of none are entitled to consideration, except the great names in medicine,
especially those who have made it the business of a life-time, to observe and study
the symptoms in the living subject, and to examine that subject after death. Abernethy says, "Can Consumption be cured? Why that is a question which a man who
was brought up in a dissecting room would laugh at—it is every day demonstrated
to him." It will be found under the proper head, that the best physicians indorse the
following strong language :—

"Pathological Anatomy has perhaps never afforded more convincing evidence in
proof of the curability of the disease, than it has in that of Tubercular Consumption!"

"The most eminent pathologists of the PRESENT day, concur in the opinion, that
PULMONARY CONSUMPTION is most certainly curable, even in the last and worst stages
of the disease." See page 127, &c. Argument on a point so palpable, is useless.

Many persons are pronounced to have "only Bronchitis," and the decision removes
immense weight from the patient's mind; yet of how many has it been written,
within a year of such decision, "died of Consumption."

Bronchitis often ends in Consumption, yet persons have died of this so called
Bronchitis, whose lungs, on examination after death, were found to be perfectly sound,
showing conclusively, that they are two distinct diseases, yet so much alike as to be
constantly confounded. It follows then, irresistibly, that the ordinary modes of deciding on any given case, whether it is Consumption or Bronchitis, are deceptive, and
ought not to be relied on. Numerous cases are recorded in medical works, where
persons on examination, are found to have died of Consumption, and yet all the
usual modes of detecting that disease, during life, failed to indicate its presence. It
is evident then, as well as universally acknowledged among medical men, that there
is needed a more infallible test of the presence of Consumption, especially in its
earliest stages, when alone its cure can be promised with any certainty. No one
denies the curable nature of Phthisis, if attempted at the very first onset of the
disease: but Stethescopy and Auscultation are confessedly unable to ascertain this
vitally important point. I believe myself to possess the means and ability to do
this, with an accuracy allied to infallibility, and with a power of conviction akin to
demonstration.

THE OBJECT OF THIS PUBLICATION IS

1. To show the difference between *Laryngitis, Bronchitis,* and *Consumption.*
2. To introduce a new and reliable method of ascertaining the existence of Consumption in its earliest stages.
3. To advocate the certainty of the prompt and permanent cure of Consumption,
when undertaken before the lungs have begun to decay, and as soon as the new diagnostic announces its first inroads on the system.
4. To recommend a new and successful mode of treating those affections of the
throat and lungs, which are *called* Bronchitis, and which are not Consumption.
5. To show that when Consumption has once fairly fixed itself in the system, and
the work of decay has already begun in the lungs, recovery is seldom to be expected,
and ought never to be promised.
6. To prove, that although recovery ought not to be promised when decay has
begun in the lungs, yet efforts ought to be made, diligent and persevering efforts for

a restoration, because such a recovery does sometimes take place, and persons die many years afterwards of some totally different disease; and the examination of the lungs after death, has most conclusively shown that a considerable portion of them had decayed away ten or fifteen years before; for case, see page 127 of 5th edition.

7· That the most eminent physicians, living and dead, clearly admit, and assert in terms as strong as language can express, (see pages 127 to 145, fifth edition,) that *recoveries from Consumption in its last stages do sometimes occur.*

These seven are the main objects held in view in this publication. In the large fifth edition of 1849 a variety of cases are given in full, showing in what way the diseases in question generally arise, progress and terminate,—showing also what kind of cases recover, and what are the predominating symptoms in each particular malady, whether Bronchitis Laryngitis or Consumption.

Having abandoned the general practice of medicine some fifteen years since, and turned my attention exclusively to the treatment of the throat and lungs, I have had perhaps, as wide a field of observation and experience as any physician in America.

In the prosecution of my inquiries, I have spent some time in England, Scotland and France, where facilities for investigating diseases are enjoyed which are not to be met with in this country.

This book is not written to instruct medical men; but in the language of the common people, that any one who can read at all, may understand it, and know what are the signs and symptoms of the diseases treated of IN THEIR FIRST STAGES, and knowing, many apply for relief in time, and thus be saved, WITH GREAT CER-TAINTY, from bitter sufferings, and a dreadful death.

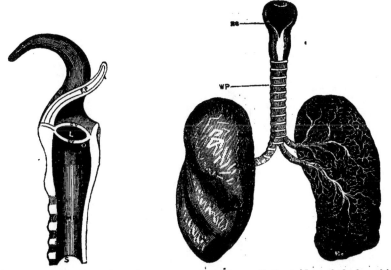

The engravings above have been prepared to give a distinct idea of the breathing apparatus, and are sufficiently accurate for that purpose.

The large figure represents the opening into the Larynx, marked R. G.

W. P. indicates the windpipe. Its natural size is about one inch in diameter.

Just below the letters W. P. are seen the three lobes of the Lungs with their covering, on the right side of the breast.

On the left side, the covering is taken off, to show how the windpipe divides off into the Bronchial branches. At the end of each one of these branches are bulbs, more distinctly seen on the upper part; these are the bronchial tubes terminating in air cells and clusters of air cells. Around the end of each bronchial extremity it is estimated by M. Rochoux, that there are grouped near eighteen thousand of these cells . and that the whole number of air cells in the Lungs, is about 170 millions; if these little air cells and bladders could be all cut open and spread out continuously, they would cover a space of twenty thousand square inches. On tracing a bronchial branch, it is found at first to be cartilaginous; it then loses this character, yet retains its perfectly circular form, having no air cells opening in to it; and lastly, the air cells increase so much in number, and open into the branches so closely to one another, that the tube can no longer retain its circular form, but becomes reduced to an irregular passage, running between the cells; and ultimately ends by forming a terminal air cell. It is only attempted in the figure to show how the bronchial branches terminate in a bulb or air cell. The rest can be imagined.

The smaller figure represents T. the Tongue; E. P. the Epiglottis; cv. cv. the upper and lower vocal chords; and W. P. Windpipe. The whole cut down in two pieces through the centre, and gives a more accurate side view of these parts than any engraving I have seen.

The egg like space, or chamber, between the vocal chords marked c.v., is called the ventricle of the Larynx, the remainder of the figure represents Windpipe. The air cells in the engraving are represented as circular, but in reality, they are irregularly shaped, the cavities having generally four or five unequal sides, just as common bladders would appear, when partially distended with air in a confined space.

TABLE OF FOOD.

NAME.	Mode of preparation	Time of digestion.	Digestibility 100 easiest.	NAME.	Mode of preparation	Time of digestion.	Digestibility 100 easiest.
Aponeurosis	boiled	3	33	Marrow, animal, spinal	boiled	2 40	37
Apples, mellow	raw	2	50	Meat and Vegetables	hashed	2 30	40
Do. sour, hard	do.	2 50	35	Milk	boiled	2	50
Do. sweet, mellow	do.	1 50	54	Do.	raw	2 15	44
Barley	boiled	2	50	Mutton, fresh	roasted	3 15	30
Bass, striped, fresh	broiled	3	33	Do. do.	broiled	3	33
Beans, pod	boiled	2 30	40	Do. do.	boiled	3	33
Do. and green corn	do.	3 45	26	Oysters, fresh	raw	2 55	34
Beef, fresh, lean, rare	roasted	3	33	Do. do.	roasted	3 15	30
Do. do. do. dry	do.	3 30	28	Do. do.	stewed	3 30	28
Do. do. steak	broiled	3	33	Parsnips	boiled	2 30	40
Do. with salt only	boiled	2 45	36	Pig, sucking	roasted	2 30	40
Do. with mustard, &c.	do.	3 30	28	Pig's feet, soused	boiled	1	100
Do.	fried	4	25	Pork, fat and lean	roasted	5 15	19
Do. old, hard salted	boiled	4 15	23	Do. recently salted	boiled	4 30	22
Beets	do.	3 45	26	Do. do.	fried	4 15	23
Brains, animal	do.	1 45	57	Do. do.	broiled	3 15	30
Bread, corn	baked	3 15	30	Do. do.	raw	3	33
Do. wheat, fresh	do.	3 30	28	Do. do.	stewed	3	33
Butter †	melted	3 30	28	Potatoes, Irish	boiled	3 30	28
Cabbage, head	raw	2 30	40	Do. do.	roasted	2 30	40
Do. with vinegar	do.	2	50	Do. do.	baked	3 20	40
Do.	boiled	4 30	22	Rice	boiled	1	100
Cake, corn	baked	3	33	Sago	do.	1 45	57
Do. sponge	do.	2 30	40	Salmon, salted	do.	4	25
Carrot, orange	boiled	3 15	30	Sausage fresh	broiled	3 20	30
Cartilage, gristle	do.	4 15	23	Soup, barley	boiled	1 30	66
Catfish, fresh	fried	3 30	28	Do. bean	do.	3	33
Cheese, old, strong	raw	3 30	28	Do. beef, vegetables, and bread	do.	4	25
Chicken, full grown	fricasseed	2 45	36	Do. chicken	do.	3	33
Codfish, cured dry	boiled	2	50	Do. marrow bones	do.	4 51	23
Corn, (green) and beans	do.	3 45	26	Do. mutton	do.	3 30	28
Custard	baked	2 45	36	Do. oyster	do.	3 30	28
Duck, domesticated	roasted	4	25	Suet, beef, fresh	do.	5 30	18
Do. wild	do.	4 30	22	Do mutton	do.	4 30	22
Dumpling, apple	boiled	3	33	Tapioca	do.	2	50
Eggs, fresh	hard boiled	3 30	28	Tendon, boiled	do.	5 30	18
Do. do.	soft boiled	3	33	Tripe, soused	do.	1	100
Do. do.	fried	3 30	28	Trout, salmon, fresh	do.	1 30	66
Do. do.	roasted	2 15	44	Do. do.	fried	1 30	66
Do. do.	raw	2	50	Turkey, domestic	roasted	2 30	40
Do. do.	whipped	1 30	66	Do. do.	boiled	2 25	51
Flounder, fresh	fried	3 30	28	Do. wild	roasted	2 18	43
Fowls, domestic	boiled	4	25	Turnips, flat	boiled	3 30	28
Do. do.	roasted	4	25	Veal, fresh	broiled	4	25
Gelatin	boiled	2 30	40	Do. do.	fried	4 30	22
Goose, wild	roasted	2 30	40	Vegetables and meat hashed	warmed	2 30	40
Hart, animal	fried	4	25	Venison, steak	broiled	135	63]
Lamb, fresh	boiled	2 30	40				
Liver, Beef's, fresh	do.	2	50				

† [In the case of oils, and other substances of similar nature, which undergo little digestion in the stomach the period merely indicates the time that elapses before they are sent into the duodenum.

PLAIN STATEMENTS.

The pulse and the breathing have a strict relation to each other, averaging seventy-two and eighteen in a minute, and in proportion as they are steadily above these, for weeks together, the person is approaching to, or is in a decline, and another symptom which invariably accompanies these, is, that as these are rapid, the lungs take in less and less air, averaging in health two hundred and twenty-two inches at a full inspiration.

A person of average physical proportions, never comes to me in the last stages of Consumption, who does not present a pulse of ninety-six and upwards, a breathing of twenty-four and upwards, and a corresponding diminution of the amount of air which his lungs should contain at a full inspiration. See case on page fifty-one and fifty-five.

Knowing, then, the conditions in health as to these three points, and the *invariable* conditions in the last stages of consumptive disease, the value of the means which detects the *very first* departures from the healthy standard, must, beyond all question, be most important and satisfactory; and the approximations from disease *back to health*, are equally valuable, so that I may use, in reference to this mode, precisely the language of the London Lancet, in reference to the *sonometer* which measures the amount of sound in the ear's return to health: "By means of this, the exact amount of hearing, (respiration,) which a patient possesses, can be measured with the greatest accuracy before the treatment commences, so that no doubt can exist as to whether the patient is relieved by the remedy."

A man may come to me, having lost a portion of his lungs by decay, and the decay is progressing, this decay cannot be arrested instantly, consequently, for a short time he will measure less and less up to the time of arresting the progress of the decay, and he will remain at that low figure, because the lungs are gone, and new ones cannot be created in their place, yet he may enjoy reasonable health for years, the *pulse and breathing being natural.* See pages 52; 675, **C.**.

In full health, he should have measured 270.

When he came to me had 244.

When he left, not needing farther advice, he had 192.

When this patient first came to me, I told him he could be saved, but never could be perfectly restored.

Again, if a small portion of the lungs is lost by decay, say a twentieth or tenth, if the patient be young, and of a good constitution otherwise, a proper course of treatment and lung exercise, will cause the remainder of the lungs to do more than their natural share, and thus that remainder be made to take in as much air as when the lungs were in a whole condition. See page 53, case **W. B.**; compare line four from the bottom with line twenty.

AN INTERESTING CALCULATION.

A tall man will take in at a full breath nine pints of air, while in ordinary breathing he takes in one pint, or forty cubic inches. If he be all at once deprived of this whole 40 inches, he will die in three minutes, and if death results from a total deprivation, an injury to health and life must take place in proportion as the amount breathed is less than forty inches; for example, of a hundred letter pressmen, working in a room having less than 500 cubic feet of air to breathe, thirteen per cent had spitting of blood induced; while as many men having more than 600 feet, gave only four per cent of spitting blood; showing that, that most fatal symptom of Consumption is brought on in proportion as men breathe less pure air than health requires; the effect being the same whether there are not lungs to receive it, or whether there be not the air to be received.

It is with food as with air; a person soon dies if wholly deprived of either, but will gradually and a long time linger, if not quite enough is given for the wants of the system; and all are familiar with the fact, that consumptives gradually die as the lungs, by decay, become less and less able to receive the due amount of air, hence my reason for keeping an eye constantly fixed on the condition and character of the breathing, *a thing almost entirely lost sight of by modern practitioners;* a physician scarcely ever calls without feeling and counting the pulse; how often has the physician, who is now reading these lines, counted the respiration of a consumptive patient!! I, however, do not rely upon counting, I measure the amount by cubic inches, leaving no ground for conjecture or for guess work; and it is by this means that I measure a patient's gradual restoration, or his gradual death, as on pages 53 and 54.

THE LUNGS

Of a common man contain about one hundred and seventy millions of little bladders, or air cells, or little holes of different sizes, as in a sponge, and if these were cut open, and spread out, they would cover a space thirty times greater than the man's skin would; over one side this vast surface the blood is spread out, by means of very small blood vessels, on the other side, the air is diffused, and the substance of these little bladders is so thin, that the blood and air, in effect, come in contact, and the result of this contact is purification, heat and life; and death is the result, if this contact is prevented for three minutes; the reader will feel, therefore, how great is the necessity for a constant and full supply of pure air to the lungs. Hence the reason that those who live out of doors the most, live the longest, other things being equal. Of the 120,000 who die every year in England and Wales of Consumption, the greater number is among in-door laborers. This is the reason too, why the families of the rich in cities, soon become extinct; in summer they stay in the house to keep out of the sun, and in the winter to keep out of the cold; their faces are pale, their skin is flabby, and their limbs are weak; a young girl is put out of breath if she runs across the street; and seldom a day passes without a complaint of a head ache or bad cold, or chilliness or want of appetite, while the old father and mother of sixty winters or more, who lived in log cabins, cutting wood, hoeing corn. building fences, mauling rails, feeding cattle, spinning flax, weaving jeans in the old loom house during the day, and knitting socks in the chimney corner at night, going to bed a little after dark, and getting up to work before day, *they* scarcely know what an ache or a pain is, can eat heartily three times a day, and are sound asleep in five minutes after the head reaches the pillow, and what is perhaps better, are always forbearing, good natured, cheerful, hospitable and kind, while their city progeny are poor, helpless, fretful, complaining invalids, heirs to millions, they may possibly live to inherit for a brief period, but never can enjoy. The remedy for this, to some extent, may be found on pages 35 and 48.

BRANDY AND THROAT DISEASE.

In several instances persons have applied to me who had been advised to take brandy freely for a throat affection. None but an ignorant man or a drunkard would give such advice; it is warranted by no one principle in medicine, reason or common sense. The throat is inflamed, the brandy inflames the whole body, and the throat affection, being less urgent from its being scattered over a larger surface, is less felt, and the excitement of the liquor gives a general feeling of wellness. until the system becomes accustomed to the stimulous, and then the throat, body and the man all the more speedily go to ruin together.

I have in my mind, while writing these lines, the melancholy history of two young men, one from Kentucky and the other from Missouri, who were advised to drink brandy freely, three times a day, for a throat complaint; one of them, within a year, became a confirmed drunkard and lost his property, and will leave an interesting family in want within another year. The other was one of the most high-minded, honorable young men I have lately known; he was the only son of a widow, and she was rich; *within six months* he became a regular toper, lost his business, spent all his money and left secretly for California many thousands of dollars in debt.

WOMEN AND THROAT AIL.

Many women have throat affections of various grades, generally the result of dyspepsia; they eat a great deal, have indigestion, a remedy being at hand, some preparation of soda, they swallow it, feel better, and next day over eat again; in due time the coats of the stomach become impaired, permanent inflammation is set up, this extends upwards to the throat, and in time takes on ulceration, ending in death.

FEVER AND AGUE.

It is believed by many that there is not much Consumption where fever and ague prevails. According to my experience, it is the very reverse. A large number of cases in my note book, are, in the opinion of the patient, traceable to fever and ague, as I always ask, " *What do you think brought on your disease?*"

IS CONSUMPTION CATCHING.

Very many widows and widowers who come to me for Consumption. say that their companions died of that disease. This is a fact; the reader can form his own opinion. My belief is, that a perfectly healthy person will not take on Consumption from intimate association with a consumptive; but if there is a scrofulous habit, or a tendency to Consumption, the same disease will be excited in a great majority of cases. When two persons are so unfavorably situated, the best guard against such a result, is a regular, temperate life, eating plain food, mostly vegetable, meat only at dinner; drinking nothing but cold water; sleeping in large, well ventilated rooms, without fire, and being out of doors at least five hours in every twenty-four, frequent washings, rubbings and scrubbings of the whole surface with cold water, warm feet and a cheerful spirit.

ASTHMA.

I have said nothing of this in these pages. It needs no description, as it consists in spells of difficult, distressing breathing, coming on generally at stated times, with intervals from a few hours to several months. When it is organic, that is arising from some injury to the structure or body of the lungs, there is no cure this side the grave.

In most instances, it is a functional disease, owing to constitutional causes, and equally excited by a cold or indigestion. Cases of this kind I have removed in a few days, and with proper care of the general health, they do not return; and if the general health is kept up long enough, to *break up the habit of Asthma*, the system is permanently relieved from the liability to it; and a very great deal is done towards effecting this desirable result by keeping the liver and bowels in a healthful condition, and adopting Sir Astly Cooper's mode of bathing.

A SUBSTITUTE FOR THE BATH.

The following plan was adopted by Sir Astly Cooper during many years of his life —and is worthy the example of those who can not enjoy the blessing of bathing in their own house.

" Immediately on rising from bed, and having all previously ready, take off your night dress, then take up from your earthern pan of two gallons of water a towel, quite wet, but not dropping; begin at your head, rubbing hair and face, and neck and ears well; then wrap yourself behind and before, from neck to chest, your arms, and every portion of your body. Remand your towel into the pan, charge it afresh with water, and repeat once all I have mentioned, excepting the head, unless that be in a heated state, when you may do so, and with advantage. Three minutes will now have elapsed. Throw your towel into the pan, and then proceed, with two coarse long towels, to scrub your head, and face, and body, front and rear, when four minutes will have you in a glow; then wash and hard rub your feet, brush your hair, and complete your toilette; and trust me that this will give new zest to your existence. A mile of walking may be added with advantage."

In addition to this, means must be taken to cause the generation of internal heat, so as to give the system the power of repelling external cold, and thus doubly guarding the asthmatic from taking cold. There are two sources of heat in the system:

The digestion of food.

The consumption of oxygen.

Then such food must be used as will eliminate most heat, and the alimentary organs kept in a condition to best digest that food; the amount of caloric eliminated is as various as the articles of food, for example:

Barley meal eliminates 68¼ per cent of the heat forming principle ;
Oat meal   ,,•   68   ,,
Wheat   ,,   62
Peas and beans ,,   51½
Potatoes   ,,   25
Carrots   ,,   10   ,,
Turnips   ,,   9   ,,

We perceive from this, that there is truth in the common remark of nurses that such and such things are heating, and others are cooling. The human body must have heat, and it is more natural that it should come from the inside than from the outside, that it should be obtained from a vigorous and healthful circulation than from heavy clothing and warm rooms, both of which, as every observer must know, have an enervating influence on both body and mind. The best mode, then, of treating Asthma, of this form, is to secure a vigorous circulation and respiration by appropriate diet and abundant exercise in a pure condensed atmosphere, and to keep this up until the system has grown out of the asthmatic habit.

CASE OF FUNCTIONAL ASTHMA.

Woman aged 40, has had Asthma at various intervals for two years, but the attacks have become so frequent of late, that the cough is almost constant, has fallen off thirty pounds, and for the last seven weeks has not lain down in bed to sleep.

I treated her on the general principles above named. The first night she slept several hours, and in a week could sleep all night lying down ; in five weeks she called to know if the asthma was permanently gone or if it would return, as she now had no cough, no pain, appetite had returned, and was gaining flesh every day. I told her if she kept up the general directions, the probability was, that she would not be troubled with it again. Whether it ever returned I cannot say, as the patient has never since called ; whether this was because it returned as bad as ever, and she became discouraged, or whether from the bill not being paid, I cannot say. From all that I have seen, it is my opinion that three-fourths of all cases of Asthma can be cured on the principles above stated ; when the Asthma has been preceded by long hepatic or dyspeptic derangement, the return to health is proportionably slow.

THROAT AIL.

I have found it of very little utility to attempt to enforce rules for the prevention of disease of any kind, especially in reference to the lungs and throat ; but as far as clergymen are concerned I here propose one or two items of observance.

Never accustom yourself to drink a drop of water, or chew or swallow a particle of more solid substances while making an address, nor immediately before, nor after.

Accustom yourself to speak in *a conversational tone,* with the same earnestness, of tone, and gesture as you employ when conversing upon an interesting subject with an attentive listener, this is the true style of real eloquence, and carries your hearers along with a quiet power, far more irresistible than a louder delivery or more frantic gesticulation. It is the still, and quiet, and subdued tone that carries with it the deepest and most lasting impression. Speaking thus, no rules are needed for the modulations of the voice, or regulation of the respiration. The most natural way of speaking, is to speak without rule ; only feel deeply the truth of what you say, and be in earnest in urging those truths, then you will never speak *loud* or *long*. No one can ever bring on throat disease, if he be guided by these principles. Speaking is a natural function, and the voice organs can no more be injured by speaking in a natural way, than the lungs can be injured by breathing: and can it ever be necessary to speak in an unnatural way? Let clergymen ponder this question well, and let them *speak* their feelings, and not *read* them.

Another observance should be—after the services are over, remain until all the congregation are gone, and still longer, if cold enough for fire ; and on leaving the door keep the mouth steadily shut, not uttering a single word until you get into a room where there is fire ; by thus sending the air to the lungs in a circuitous way, by the nostrils, it is somewhat warmed before it reaches the throat and lungs, and two sudden shocks are prevented, first in going out into the cold air from the church, and next coming into a warm room. If the weather is very cold, a handkerchief should be held over the nose, so that the air expired may mingle to a certain extent with the air about to be inspired, and warm it a little.

After speaking in a room where there is fire, or in one a little warmer than outdoors, never ride home, always walk, and walk very briskly until the blood begins to circulate freely; if you live too far off to walk, remain an hour or so with a neighbor before you start; the object is to prevent a feeling of chilliness running over you even for an instant.

In the course of my life, I have had occasion to speak two or three times a day for weeks together in close, crowded, heated rooms, in the depth of winter, and sometimes to go a mile or two to a resting place, and never once during these occasions. caught a cold, or had hoarseness or sore throat. I speak from experience and not theory. Believe truly, feel deeply and speak sincerely, and there never will be any need of a long speech, a loud speech, or one that *shall strain the voice*, or produce Throat Ail.

SLEEP.

Sound, connected, early, refreshing sleep, is as essential to health as our daily food. There is no merit in simply getting up early. The full amount of sleep requisite for the wants of the system should be obtained even if it requires till noon. I go to bed at nine o'clock the year round, and I stay there until I feel rested; but I do not go to sleep again after I have once awaked of myself, after daylight. I remain in bed until the feeling of tiredness goes off, if there is any, and I get up when I feel like it. I do not sleep in the day-time; it is a pernicious practice, and always diminishes the soundness of repose at night. Dr. Holyoke, after he was a hundred years old, said, "I have always taken care to have a full proportion of sleep, which, I suppose, has contributed to my longevity." The want of sufficient sleep is a frequent cause of insanity. To obtain good sleep, the mind should be in a sober, quiet frame for several hours before bed-time. I think people require one hour's more sleep in winter than in summer. In connection with this subject, the North British Review illustrates the importance of sufficient sleep on a parallel with the natural history of the Sabbath:—"The Creator has given us a natural restorative—sleep; and a moral restorative—Sabbath keeping; and it is ruin to dispense with either. Under the pressure of high excitement, individuals have passed weeks together with little sleep or none; but when the process is long continued, the over-driven powers rebel, and fever, delirium and death come on. Nor can the natural amount be systematically curtailed without corresponding mischief. The Sabbath does not arrive like sleep. The day of rest does not steal over us like the hour of slumber. It does not entrance us almost, whether we will or not; but, addressing us as intelligent beings, our Creator assures us that we need it, and bids us notice its return, and court its renovation. And if, going in the face of the Creator's kindness, we force ourselves to work all days alike, it is not long till we pay the forfeit. The mental worker—the man of business, or the man of letters—finds his ideas coming turbid and slow; the equipoise of his faculties is upset, he grows moody, fitful and capricious; and with his mental elasticity broken, should any disaster occur, he subsides into habitual melancholy, or in self-destruction speeds his guilty exit from a   world. And the manual worker—the artisan, the engineer—toiling on from day to day, and week to week, the bright intuition of his eyes gets blunted; and, forgetful of their cunning, his fingers no longer perform their feats of twinkling agility, nor by a plastic and tuneful touch, mold dead matter, or wield mechanic power; but mingling his life's blood in his daily drudgery, his locks are prematurely gray, his genial humor sours, and slaving it till he has become a morose or reckless man, for any extra effort, or any blink of balmy feelings. he must stand indebted to opium or alcohol."

A sleeping room should be large and airy, the higher from the ground the better, even in the country; it should contain but very little furniture, no curtains or clothing of any description should be hung up in it, nor should it contain for a moment, any vegetables or fruit, or flowers or standing liquors of any kind; nor should there be any carpet on the floor, except a small strip at the side of the bed, so that in getting out of bed a shock may not be imparted by the warm feet coming in contact with the cold floor. The fire-place should be always left open during the day for several hours; the windows and doors should be left open while the sun is shining, but the windows should be closed an hour or more before sun-down. As soon as a person is dressed in the morning, he should leave his chamber; the bedding should be hung on chairs and allowed to air for several hours. A cheerful walk of half an hour or more should then be taken before breakfast.

On going to bed, a window should be hoisted several inches at bottom, and if practicable, be let down as much at top, that while the beavy fresh air comes in below, the light and foul air may pass out above. As a general rule, it is far best to sleep in rooms where no fire has been burning since breakfast, but there should be bed-clothing enough to keep from feeling chilly. If it is bitter cold weather with high winds, it may be better to build a moderate fire about dark, but not to let it go entirely out before morning. If there is any fire at all in a sleeping room, it should not be allowed to go out altogether.

A person should sleep in one garment, a coarse cotton shirt, and no more, without a button, or pin, or string about him. No one who pretends to common cleanliness should sleep in a garment worn during the day; nor wear during the day a garment in which he has slept; any garment worn should have six or eight hours' airing every twenty-four hours.

SLEEPING APARTMENTS.

No sleeping room should be less than eight feet high, nor should it contain for each person sleeping in it, less than one hundred and fifty feet superficial measure, or about twelve feet square.

To show what a bearing a small deficiency in the action of the lungs has on the health, I present the following calculation applied to a night's sleep of eight hours:-- A person in good health and of medium size will, in that eight hours' sleep, breathe nine hundred gallons of air; but if one-fifth of his lungs are inoperative, he consumes in the same time one hundred and eighty gallons less, and in the course of twenty-four hours, seven hundred gallons less than he ought to do. No wonder then that when the lungs begin to work less freely than they ought to do, the face so soon begins to pale, the appetite fails, the strength declines, the flesh fades, and the victim dies. Not only are consumptions traceable to this habitual deficiency of respiration, but rheumatism, colds, chills, ague, bilious, yellow and putrid fevers, suppressions, whites, dyspepsia and the like. So that in every view of the case, any method which secures the prompt detection of this insufficient breathing and rectifies it without delay, should merit and demands the immediate investigation of every lover of the health and happiness of human kind.

REFLECTION AND EXAMINATION SOLICITED.

Many persons dismiss the whole subject of Consumption in a very summary manner by saying, " *it cannot be cured, and it is scarcely worth while to try.*" BUT IS THIS TRUE? *How do you know? Do you understand the nature of the disease? Have you made any investigation on the subject? Is it right to assert a thing as true, merely because you believe it to be true, without having investigated the subject thoroughly?* When a man makes a broad assertion about anything, the presumption is, that from having examined it well, he knows what he says and has a right to say it. Very many persons have a habit of uttering things in a very decided manner, but on investigation it is found that it was merely an impression which happened to strike them forcibly as true, without their having any special reason for believing it, and in many instances they cannot even tell why they believe it. It is in this way that many serious errors are extensively propagated, and their eradication becomes the work of years. It is the mark of true greatness to utter opinions modestly, even upon subjects studied for half a life-time. A great wrong is done to truth and to the world in stating what is not known to be true.

Instead, then, of statements made ignorantly and at random, I present here a statement of facts derived from the records of the hospital for Consumption in London for the last year.

1 Consumptive persons, male and female, are more inclined to marry early than others.

2 Of all who enter the hospital, counting those who were dying when they entered the door, the number leaving it improved, or not worse, was double the number of hose who got worse, or died.

3 Four and a quarter per cent. perfectly recovered, leaving the hospital without any sign of any disease whatever.

4. More men got perfectly well, than women.

5. All those who got worse had actual decay of the lungs when they entered.

6. All who had not reached the softening of tubercles, or the decaying stage, either improved or were prevented from getting worse.

7. Improvement is more probable than the reverse, even where an excavation exists.

8. The longer a person has been sick, the greater his chance for improvement.

9. Those have a greater chance of getting well whose occupations are pursued out of doors.

10. Country patients, on an average, have a slightly stronger chance of improvement than city residents.

11. Eighty-one out of every hundred had spitting of blood to a greater or less extent.

12. The first hemorrhage is apt to be most profuse.

13. Spitting of blood occurs oftenest in persons who are in the second and third stages of Consumption, especially in males.

14. In upwards of half the cases of notable hemorrhage, that is eight table-spoonfulls or more, this occurs as the first symptom.

☞ *When persons spit* blood from the lungs I have *nearly always* found it to be a sign of Consumption *in its advanced stages*, although no cough had ever *been noticed: and expectoration of blood in any form* justifies the suspicion that latent tubercles exist.

15. The importance of spitting of blood as a symptom of Consumption is extreme, even when the expectoration is simply streaked or tinged with red.

16. Males who spit blood are more apt to die than females who spit blood.

There is no doubt in my own mind, that every year the proper treatment of Consumption is better understood, and that in time it will be allowed to be one of the manageable diseases—this will be hastened in proportion as people can be induced to study the symptoms of the disease in its first approaches. From the advances constantly making in chemical science, in physiology and hygiene, better and more rational views are being taken in reference to Consumption and its treatment. Under the old plan of treatment, Blisters, Bleeding, Purging, Dieting, Confinement, men have continued to die by millions, but an entire revolution is taking place.

1. Instead of bleeding, and thus reducing the strength and the amount of blood, I take means to give more blood.

2. Instead of purging, I take every means to prevent it.

3. Instead of living on a small allowance of food, I endeavor, in every manner possible, to make them eat more and digest it better.

4. Instead of blisters and running sores, I heal them up and direct the drains through the natural channel.

5. Instead of stopping the cough, I let it alone, and in some instances promote it.

6. Instead of keeping my patients in the house I compel them to be out of doors.

7. Instead of sending them to a warm and weakening climate, I send them to a cold and bracing one, dry and still.

8. Instead of pulling down, I build up.

9. Instead of giving medicine, (in cases of simple, uncomplicated Consumption,) I prevent its use.

I throw out these hints for the use of educated medical men, to many of whom I am placed under obligations for superintending my cases at a distance, and for other civilities, therefore I have given advice to such without charge, and have done it freely, that is to those who are engaged in the practice of medicine, and are dependent on such practice for a support; this applies only to those who have never given their names countenance or encouragement in any way to secret remedies or patent contrivances for the alleviation of human suffering.

INDEX OF CONTENTS.

there is no remedy, and death is inevitable, because there the windpipe branches off nearly square, and the ulcerated part cannot be reached. Various agents are applied, such as solutions of sulphate of alum, sulphate of iron, sulphate of copper, and the nitrates, principally of silver.

As I wrote you fifteen months ago, that you had *not* Consumption, although yourself and friends believed it, I will only add on that subject, that I am joined by the most distinguished medical men living, in believing it to be a curable disease ; and I think that I have cured many cases, some of them far advanced; —of which see the fifth edition of my publication on Diseases of the Throat and Lungs, just issued. The reason that so many die of Consumption, is because they will not awake to the fact of its existence, until the lungs are already decaying, and the constitution is broken down. I wish it was generally understood that Consumption always gives a timely warning. The object in publishing my work is to explain to the community what the symptoms are, that indicate the first approaches of this, very properly, dreaded disease ; and to show how easily these symptoms could be removed, if judicious efforts were employed, as soon as the first made their appearance.

My whole medical experience for twelve or fifteen years past, and the observations which I have made in this country, and in the Hospitals and Infirmaries of Europe, confirm me in the conviction that common Consumption always begins—

By accelerated arterial action.

By accelerated respiration.

By consequent progressive debility.

By a slight cough, which usually makes its first appearance on getting up in the morning, and then on going to bed at night. The cough and pain, however, are sometimes not observable, until within four or five weeks of death.

The great point so ardently desired by medical men all over the world, has been to ascertain when Consumption was first begining its inroads on the system. The introduction of the stethescope, by the immortal Laennec, was at first hailed as the harbinger of good things in this respect. It has failed. It is universally admitted that it does not indicate the early presence of tubercles, which are the seeds of the disease; and the old treatment of Consumption, on *general principles,* was resumed, to wit: by Blisters, Setons, Issues, Nauseants and other weakening remedies, only to meet with the uniform failure of the last hundred years.

For the Consumption itself, I administer but little medicine; debility is an unfailing characteristic, and whatever increases that debility, necessarily hastens death ; and confinement to the house accelerates a like result. I seldom use the stethescope. My finger tells me of the pulse ; the ear points out a cavity, dry or partially filled with decaying and decayed lung substance, or directs to the spot where there is condensation or infiltration. But I do not rely on any one, nor any half dozen of these symptoms. I measure, in addition, in a manner infallible, the amount of air a person's lungs contain. I know, by thousands of examinations, made by myself and others, the quantity which any one of a given age, height and weight, and in undisputed health, ought to contain; and as soon as there is a fixed decrease of capacity, of five, ten or fifteen degrees ; just so soon, other things considered, I judge the person in question *"going into a decline,"* and use every effort to increase the capacity to a healthy standard, and this can be done with a frequency allied to infallibility, if attempted at the early commencement of the decline : and the chances for recovery decrease, in proportion as the patient has allowed his capacity of lungs to decrease before application.

My patients can test their improvement from week to week, and nothing is left to the physician's flattery, or their own more deceptive feelings. I have known persons in a decline, to assert from week to week, that they were better, even until within a day or two of death—but here delusions of this kind are impossible, and as soon as I perceive an established decrease in the vital capacity despite of all that I can do, I communicate the fact, and let consequences take care of themselves. Hence, when I am applied to for an opinion of a case, I give such an one as I feel to be true, without regard to my own sympathies, or the wishes of the patient or his friends. Deception in such cases, never did, and never can eventuate in true good, either to the patient or practitioner.

With these remarks, I desire to be

Very respectfully, yours.

TO CLERGYMEN AND PUBLIC SPEAKERS.

FOOD.—Its time of Digestion, easiness of Digestion, and tiveness. See table of, in the last page.

DR. HALL, 127 *Canal Street, New Orleans.* Office hours from 9 till 1 only, sively for Diseases of the Throat and Lungs, from Nov. 1st. to May 15th.

Any protracted ailment, causing hecking, hemming, hoarseness. &c., which Consumption, is *called* 'Bronketis,' (Bronchitis,) and a person having these sym feels great relief when assured that he has "only Bronchitis." But every rende remember the name of some friend, who, not very long ago, was said to have this disease, and yet has already "died of Consumption;" this fact proves either very difficult to distinguish these diseases, or that they are one and the same they cannot be the same disease, since persons who have died of Bronchitis times found on examination, to have lungs sound and whole in every part. that Bronchitis affects one side of the throat and neck more than the other when Consumption follows Bronchitis, it is *always* observed on the same side, most conclusively that Bronchitis, unarrested, usually ends in Consumption; so generally the case, that distinguished medical writers have asserted that Con is the cause of Bronchitis, and must have existed before the Bronchitis appear latter term is used in this article to mean the same as Throat Ail, Clergyman's Sore and Chronic Laryngitis, although it is not really so. This Laryngitis, or Throa answers to a spot about Adam's Apple, or under the jaws, and gives rise to fre hemming, hecking, clearing the throat, swallowing, hoarseness, loss of voice; goi to produce a constant harrassing cough, weariness, depression of spirits, falling off ing across the breast, difficulty of breathing, spitting of blood, night sweats, and I have detected this sore spot, and by the application of mineral and metallic salts out, in some instances, giving any internal medicine, have removed *permanently* all symptoms within a fortnight—but usually it requires weeks, and sometimes mon persevering applications.

"Consumption can't be cured," is an expression uttered with great positivenes, most so, by those who are in robust health, and who feel quite sure that they hav symptoms of the disease; at the same time, intelligent physicians of all countries ily admit that it may be averted with great certainty, if attempted at the first on the malady; but the great misfortune hitherto has been, that no means were known would certainly detect the presence of the disease, except in its advanced, and co quently incurable stages; it is now universally acknowledged, that Auscultation and Stet scopy are inadequate to its early detection; any mode therefore, which promises to r this important defect, should engage the attention, and secure the investigation of all good. I believe, not only that this can be done, but that it is already reduced to ence—the science of "PULMOMETRY," or *Lung Measurement*, which *demonstrates* following important points:

Whether the lungs are sound, whole, and free from consumptive disease.

Whether it is Consumption, or only Bronchitis.

If Consumption, what proportion of the lungs, are inoperative, by reason of colla solidification, infiltration, or actual decay.

And last, though not least, the important question whether the patient is getting ter or worse, is not left to be decided by the physician's wishes, or the patient's fallacious hopes, but by a sterner test, which admits of no bribe, and knows no tery.

It not only distinguishes between consumption and bronchitis, but points out the tence of the former disease in its very first faint beginnings—and more, it reaches ba the point where there is no actual consumption, but only the preparing of the sy for taking on that justly dreaded disease; and if these early indications were but he and judicious means were promptly employed, they would seldom fail to avert the rible scourge, and one would not die of consumption, where great numbers now di I greatly desire that these things should be known from one border of our contin the other, for I believe the lives of many might be saved thereby.

I have no secrets in my practice, and never had any, except that of taking up a si branch of medicine, giving it my exclusive attention, and always keeping this fact be the people, and I am satisfied with the result. I graduated many years ago in the A pathic or Old School of medicine, and have adhered to its principles to this hour, they have gained upon my confidence and respect ever since. [☞See my last publi tion, fifth edition, with additions and engravings, 214 pages 8vo., bound in mnsli paper; sold at No, 14 Camp st., New Orleans, by J. B. Steele; and at No. 12 W Fourth st., Cincinnati, by J. D. Thorpe.